Interpretation of Emergency Head CT

A practical handbook

Second Edition

T0201628

Interpretation of Emergency Head CT

A practical handbook

Second Edition

Erskine J. Holmes, MRCS, FCEM, CFEU
Consultant in Emergency Medicine
Craigavon Area Hospital, Southern Trust, Northern Ireland

Rakesh R. Misra, BSc (Hons), FRCS (Eng), FRCR
Consultant Radiologist, Wycombe Hospital
Buckinghamshire Healthcare NHS Trust

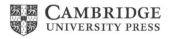
CAMBRIDGE
UNIVERSITY PRESS

CAMBRIDGE
UNIVERSITY PRESS

University Printing House, Cambridge CB2 8BS, United Kingdom

One Liberty Plaza, 20th Floor, New York, NY 10006, USA

477 Williamstown Road, Port Melbourne, VIC 3207, Australia

314-321, 3rd Floor, Plot 3, Splendor Forum, Jasola District Centre, New Delhi - 110025, India

103 Penang Road, #05-06/07, Visioncrest Commercial, Singapore 238467

Cambridge University Press is part of the University of Cambridge.

It furthers the University's mission by disseminating knowledge in the pursuit of education, learning and research at the highest international levels of excellence.

www.cambridge.org
Information on this title: www.cambridge.org/9781107495937
10.1017/9781316178881

© E. J. Holmes and R. R. Misra 2017

This publication is in copyright. Subject to statutory exception and to the provisions of relevant collective licensing agreements, no reproduction of any part may take place without the written permission of Cambridge University Press.

First published 2009
Second edition 2017
Reprinted 2022

Printed in Great Britain by Ashford Colour Press Ltd.

A catalogue record for this publication is available from the British Library

Library of Congress Cataloguing in Publication data
Names: Holmes, Erskine J., author. | Misra, Rakesh R., author.
Title: Interpretation of emergency head CT : a practical handbook / Erskine J. Holmes, Rakesh R. Misra.
Other titles: Interpretation of emergency head computed tomography
Description: Second edition. | Cambridge, United Kingdom ; New York : Cambridge University Press, 2016. | Includes bibliographical references and index.
Identifiers: LCCN 2016058545 | ISBN 9781107495937 (alk. paper)
Subjects: | MESH: Brain – diagnostic imaging | Head – diagnostic imaging | Radiography | Emergencies | Tomography, X-Ray Computed | Handbooks
Classification: LCC RC349.R3 | NLM WL 39 | DDC 616.8/047572–dc23
LC record available at https://lccn.loc.gov/2016058545

ISBN 978-1-107-49593-7

Cambridge University Press has no responsibility for the persistence or accuracy of URLs for external or third-party internet websites referred to in this publication, and does not guarantee that any content on such websites is, or will remain, accurate or appropriate.

....

Every effort has been made in preparing this book to provide accurate and up-to-date information which is in accord with accepted standards and practice at the time of publication. Although case histories are drawn from actual cases, every effort has been made to disguise the identities of the individuals involved. Nevertheless, the authors, editors and publishers can make no warranties that the information contained herein is totally free from error, not least because clinical standards are constantly changing through research and regulation. The authors, editors and publishers therefore disclaim all liability for direct or consequential damages resulting from the use of material contained in this book. Readers are strongly advised to pay careful attention to information provided by the manufacturer of any drugs or equipment that they plan to use.

Dedicated to my parents, Sally and Erskine Holmes, for making me the person I am today. **E. J. H.**

Dedicated to my late mother, Darshan Misra. You sacrificed so much to allow me to grow into the person I am. **R. R. M.**

Contents

Preface

Welcome to the second edition of *Interpretation of Emergency Head CT*.

The aim of this book is again to prepare interested specialists with a structured, image-driven handbook for CT Head and Neck interpretation. With the advances and refinement of imaging protocols in trauma, we felt it was time to include guidance on trauma CT neck interpretation. A schema is provided by which to analyse the images, in order to develop greater confidence in diagnosing the most common and time-critical problems. Up-to-date images, with accompanying text, make this book an accessible reference and aide-memoire for medical and allied professionals. The topics included should be useful for anybody revising for postgraduate examinations, and it should also prove to be an invaluable text for medical and radiography students alike. Small enough to carry around, we hope that we have once again provided a reliable reference for use anytime, regardless of the time of day or night.

Acknowledgement

Thank you to Dr Jonathan Morrow, ED physician in training, for his time and valuable contribution to the new edition.

Abbreviations

ACom	Anterior communicating
ADC	Apparent diffusion coefficient
APTT	Activated partial thromboplastin time
AVM	Arteriovenous malformation
BP	Blood pressure
CCF	Congestive cardiac failure
CPP	Cerebral perfusion pressure
CSF	Cerebrospinal fluid
CT	Computer tomography
CTV	CT venogram
CVA	Cerebrovascular accident
DWI	Diffusion-weighted imaging
ECA	External carotid artery
ECG	Electrocardiogram
EDH	Extradural haemorrhage
ETA	Estimated time of arrival
ETT	Endotracheal tube
FB	Frontal bone
GCS	Glasgow Coma Scale
GI	Gastrointestinal
HII	Hypoxic–ischaemic injury
HR	Heart rate
HU	Hounsfield Unit
ICA	Internal carotid artery
ICP	Intracranial pressure
i.m.	Intramuscular
INR	International normalised ratio
i.v.	Intravenous
LP	Lumbar puncture
M:F	Male:female
MCA	Middle cerebral artery
MR	Magnetic resonance
MRI	Magnetic resonance imaging
NICE	National Institute of Clinical Excellence
OB	Occipital bone
PACS	Patient Archive and Communication System
PB	Parietal bone
PCom	Posterior communicating
RIND	Reversible ischaemic neurological deficit
RR	Respiratory rate
SAH	Subarachnoid haemorrhage
SDH	Subdural haematoma

SLE	Systemic lupus erythematosus
SSS	Superior sagittal sinus
STB	Squamous temporal bone
TB	Tuberculosis
TIA	Transient ischaemic attack
WCC	White cell count

Introduction

Computer tomography (CT) is now routinely being used 24 hours a day, 7 days a week in the trauma setting. CT is often the initial imaging modality of choice; not only for diagnosis, but also to guide treatment.

The most common request for CT out of hours is brain imaging. In the trauma patient a protocol-driven CT cervical spine is now commonly performed alongside the CT brain.

CT is a vital tool in the assessment of patients with serious head injury. It remains the investigation of choice for the assessment of acute haemorrhage and bony injury. Consequently, patient management has been transformed since its inception, as rapid imaging and diagnosis of intracranial pathology can facilitate emergency intervention. Equally, a delay in diagnosis, and treatment, may adversely affect outcome and prognosis.

Patients' expectations of modern medical technology are high. There are ever-increasing time pressures to form rapid diagnoses, and improve efficiency, in the face of a more litigious society. The European Working Time Directive is likely to make doctors feel more vulnerable, with shift patterns reducing personal experience and training opportunities.

Furthermore, the multidisciplinary team on duty in the Hospital at Night Scheme may not possess the appropriate expertise between them to interpret emergency imaging. Yet, the NICE guidelines are in place to further increase the number of CT scans performed out of hours. To add to this, the nationwide shortage of Radiologists results in a limited CT service available out of hours. Hence we have the dilemma of how to provide an adequate emergency imaging service coupled with who will interpret the images.

The Royal College of Emergency Medicine has stipulated that Specialist Registrars in Emergency Medicine are expected to be able to diagnose brain pathology from CT scans of the head. Currently, in many hospitals around the country it is routine for CT head scans, performed out of hours, to be interpreted by the requesting doctor. This is likely to be a progressive future trend, with a variety of speciality groups needing to acquire these skills.

Analogous to this is electrocardiogram (ECG) interpretation; originally the domain of the Cardiologist, this is now a routine general investigation interpreted by most clinicians. It is not inconceivable that medical students, and junior medical staff alike, may need to acquire the basic skills to analyse CT abnormalities in the future, if we are to keep pace with the ever-increasing demand.

The purpose of this book is to provide a systematic approach by which to interpret and provisionally report head CT scans, based on learning to recognise common pathologies from an archive of representative images.

CT cervical spine interpretation is likely to become more commonplace in the future, as protocol-driven CT cervical spine replaces plain X-rays. Individual physicians will need to decide if provisional interpretation will be part of their clinical skill set. To facilitate this, we have provided schema for provisional interpretation.

Fundamentals of Computer Tomography Imaging

History

- In the early 1970s, Sir Godfrey Hounsfield's research produced the first clinically useful computed tomography (CT) scans.
- Original scanners took approximately 6 minutes to perform a rotation (one slice) and 20 minutes to reconstruct (Fig. 1a). Despite many technological advances since then, the principles remain the same.
- On early scanners, the tube rotated around a stationary patient, with the table moving to enable a further acquisition. The machine rotated clockwise and counter-clockwise as power was supplied via a cable.
- Modern-day helical or spiral scanners obtain power via slip ring technology, thus allowing continuous tube rotation as the patient moves through the scanner automatically (Fig. 1b). This allows a volume of data to be acquired in a single rotation, with the benefits of faster scanning, faster patient throughput and reduced patient movement artefacts.
- New multi-slice scanners use existing helical scanning technology, but have multiple rows of detectors to acquire multiple slices per tube rotation. The faster imaging with multi-slice scanners allows a larger volume of coverage and multiphase scanning during intravenous contrast administration (Fig. 2). This, coupled with improved spatial resolution, allows organ-specific as well as vascular assessment, leading to the advent of CT angiography and virtual endoscopy.
- Advanced computer processing power allows reconstructive techniques, such as three-dimensional and multiplane reformatting, providing us with additional tools with which to improve diagnostic accuracy and aid clinical management.

Technical Details

- The X-ray tube produces a narrow fan-shaped beam of collimated X-rays, which pass through the patient to reach a bank of detectors opposite the source (Fig. 3).
- X-rays are attenuated differentially by the patient, depending on the tissues through which they pass. Low-density tissues such as fat/aerated lung absorb fewer X-rays, allowing more to reach the detector. The opposite is true for dense tissues such as bone.
- The amount of transmitted X-ray radiation received by the detector provides information about the density of the tissue through which it has passed.

(a)

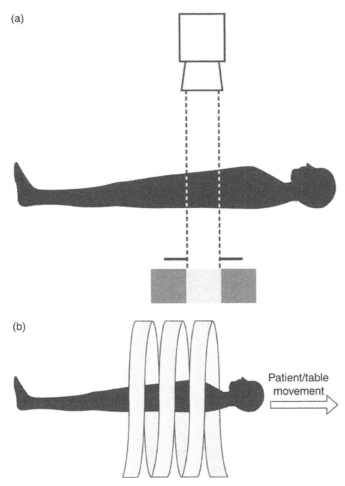

(b)

Patient/table movement

Figure 1 Diagrams showing (a) a single-slice scanning system and (b) a single-slice helical CT scanning system, where the X-ray tube continues to rotate as the patient moves through at a constant rate.

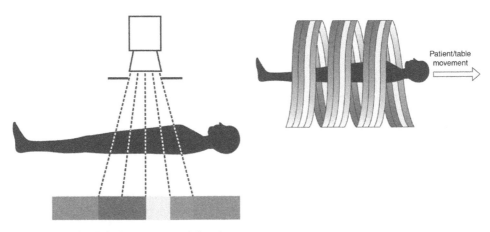

Patient/table movement

Figure 2 Multi-slice helical CT scanner with four detectors.

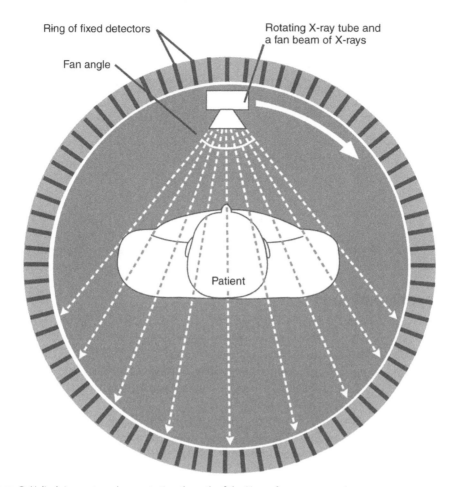

Figure 3 Helical ring system demonstrating the path of the X-rays from source to detector.

- A CT slice is divided up into a matrix of squares, e.g. 256 × 256, 512 × 512 and 1024 × 1024. The slice thickness determines the volume of these squares; these are called voxels. Using mathematical calculations, the degree to which a tissue absorbs radiation within each voxel, *the linear attenuation coefficient*, μ, is calculated and assigned a value related to the average attenuation of the tissues within it ≡ *the CT number or Hounsfield Unit (HU)*.
- Each value of μ is assigned a grey-scale value on the display monitor and is presented as a square picture element (pixel) on the image.
- Spiral scanners acquire a volume of information from which an axial slice is reconstructed, as above, using computer technology. Slices are created from data during the reconstruction phase.
- *Pitch* is defined as the distance moved by the table in millimetres, during one complete rotation of the X-ray tube, divided by the slice thickness in millimetres. In general, increasing pitch (increase table speed with a fixed slice thickness) reduces radiation dose to the patient (Fig. 4). This in turn reduces the amount of radiation reaching the detector

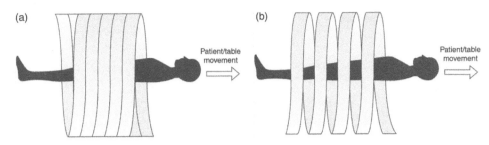

Figure 4 Low pitch vs. high pitch: (a) low-pitch scanning with the table moving less for each tube revolution, resulting in a sharper image; (b) higher-pitch scanning, resulting in stretching of the helix as the table moves more for each revolution, leading to a loss of image quality.

for interpretation, with the net result of reduced image resolution. A compromise usually exists between limiting patients' radiation dose and diagnostic image quality.

Windowing and Grey-scale

- Modern CT scanners are able to differentiate in excess of 2000 CT numbers; however, the human eye can only differentiate around 30 shades of grey.
- To maximise the perception of medically important features, images can be digitally processed to meet a variety of clinical requirements.
- The grey-scale values assigned to process CT numbers on a display monitor can be adjusted to suit special application requirements.
- Contrast can be enhanced by assigning just a narrow interval of CT numbers to the entire grey-scale on the display monitor; this is called the window technique. The range of CT numbers displayed on the whole grey-scale is called *the window width* and the average value called *the window level*.
- Changes in window width alter contrast, and changes in window level select the structure of interest to be displayed on the grey-scale, i.e. from black to white.
- Narrowing the window compresses the grey-scale to enable better differentiation of tissues within the chosen window. For example, in assessment of CT of the head, a narrow window of approximately 80 HU is used, with the centre at 30 HU. CT numbers above 70 (i.e. 30 + 40 HU) will appear white and those below –10 (i.e. 30 – 40 HU) will appear black. This allows subtle differences in tissue densities to be identified.
- Conversely, if the window were widened to 1500 HU, then each detectable shade of grey would cover 50 HU and soft tissue differentiation would be lost; however, bone/soft tissue interfaces would be apparent.
- In practical terms, the window width and level are preset on the workstation and can be adjusted by choosing the appropriate setting, i.e. a window setting for brain, posterior fossa, bone, etc.

Tissue Characteristics and Contrast Medium

- Unlike conventional radiography, CT has relatively good contrast resolution and can therefore differentiate between tissues which vary only slightly in density (Fig. 5). This is

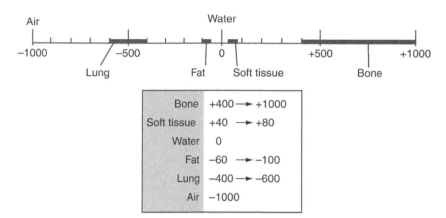

Figure 5 Graphical representation showing Hounsfield scale and CT numbers for different types of tissue, water and air.

extremely valuable when assessing the brain, as grey and white matter vary only slightly in density.

- Artefacts aside, the densest structure in the head is bone, appearing white on CT. This is followed by acute haematoma, which is denser than flowing blood, due to clot retraction and loss of water. Blood is thought to be hyperdense due to the relative density of the haemoglobin molecule. With time, blood appears isodense and then hypodense, compared to brain parenchyma, due to clot resorption. Rebleeding and layering of blood (haematocrit effect due to gravity) can often cause confusion.
- Brain can be differentiated into grey and white matter due to the difference in fatty myelin content between the two. Typically white matter (higher fatty myelin content: HU_30) is darker than the adjacent grey matter (HU_40).
- Fat and air have low attenuation values near to HU_0 and can be readily identified.
- Cerebrospinal fluid (CSF) has a similar attenuation value to water, appearing black.
- Pathological processes may become apparent due to oedema within, or adjacent to, an abnormality. Oedema is less dense than normal brain.
- Occasionally the use of a contrast medium will reveal an abnormality either due to the inherent vascular nature of a lesion or due to alteration in the normal blood–brain barrier.
- Tumours may be very variable in their appearance, but may be hyperdense due to a high nuclear/cytoplasmic ratio or tumour calcification.

Image Artefacts

- An artefact is a visual impression in the image of a feature that does not actually exist in the tissue being imaged. They are important to recognise so as not to be confused with pathology. Artefacts may occur due to scanner malfunction, patient movement and the presence of extrinsic objects within the slice being scanned, e.g. a metallic foreign body.
- Fortunately, many artefacts have now been reduced or eliminated by advances in CT speed and technology.

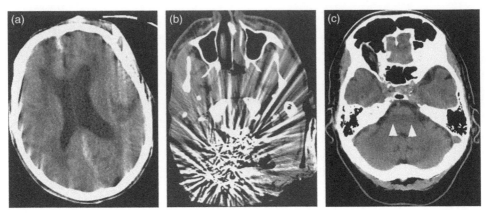

Figure 6 (a) Axial image of the brain demonstrating blurred outlines and streak pattern across the brain parenchyma secondary to movement artefacts. (b) Axial image of the brain demonstrating a star-shaped, high-density streak across the brain parenchyma secondary to metallic artefacts. (c) Axial image of the brain demonstrating bands of low attenuation across the pons secondary to beam-hardening artefacts from the skull base (arrowheads).

Movement Artefacts

- Occur with voluntary and involuntary patient motion.
- Result in streak patterns (Fig. 6a).
- Can be reduced by patient cooperation, quicker scan times and software compensation.

Partial Volume Artefacts

- The CT number reflects the average attenuation within the voxel and thus, if a highly attenuating structure is present within the voxel, it will raise the average attenuation of the whole voxel.
- Contamination can occur especially with thicker slices and near bony prominences. Always review the slices above and below to assess for structures likely to cause partial volume artefacts.
- Can be reduced by using thinner slices (e.g. posterior fossa) and software compensation.

Metallic Artefacts

- The attenuation coefficient of metal is much greater than any structure within the body. As a result, radiation is completely attenuated by the object and information about adjacent structures is lost.
- Produces characteristic star-shaped streak artefacts (Fig. 6b).
- Can be reduced by widening the window; at a cost to parenchymal detail.
- Software manipulation may help.

Beam Hardening Artefacts

- Results from an increase in the average energy of the X-ray beam as it passes through a tissue.
- Think of CT as using a spectrum of radiation energy; low-energy radiation is filtered out by high-density structures such as bone, leaving higher-energy radiation that is less absorbed by soft tissues, causing low-attenuation streak artefact.
- Characterised by linear bands of low attenuation connecting two areas of high density, such as bone, e.g. the posterior fossa in the brain (Fig. 6c).
- Can be reduced by using a filter to adjust the spectrum of radiation and by post-processing software.

Quantum Mottle

- Image reconstruction in CT requires a sufficient number of radiation photons to strike the detectors.
- The following reduce the number of radiation photons, resulting in a photon poor imaging technique, which produces a grainy CT image:
  - Reducing slice thickness to reduce partial volume artefact.
  - Alteration of CT X-ray technique to reduce the patient's radiation exposure.
  - Patient's body habitus limiting penetration of the photons.
- Quantum mottle can be reduced by increasing the slice thickness, or increasing the energy of the photon, which will increase artefact and the patient's radiation dose, respectively. A compromise between image quality, presence of artefact and radiation dose is therefore necessary.

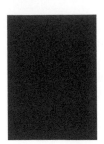

Important Anatomical Considerations

Review of Normal Axial Anatomy
Key for cerebral anatomy

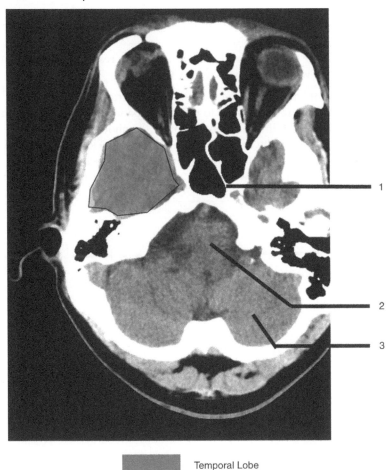

Temporal Lobe

Figure 7

1 = Sphenoid sinus
2 = Medulla oblongata
3 = Cerebellum

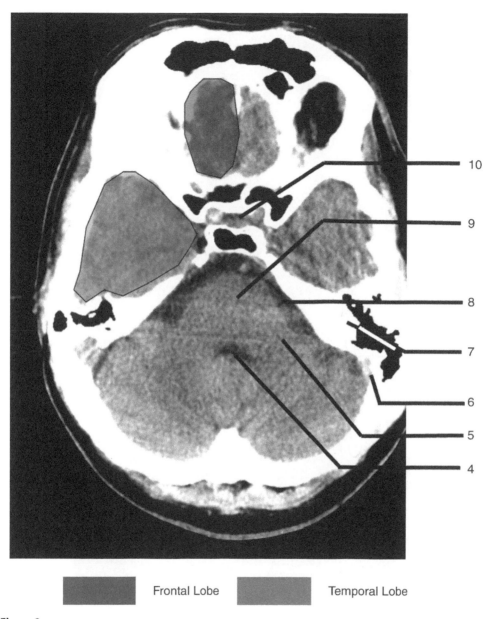

Frontal Lobe   Temporal Lobe

Figure 8

4 = Fourth ventricle
5 = Middle cerebellar peduncle
6 = Sigmoid sinus
7 = Petrous temporal bone and mastoid air cells
8 = Cerebellopontine angle
9 = Pons
10 = Pituitary fossa

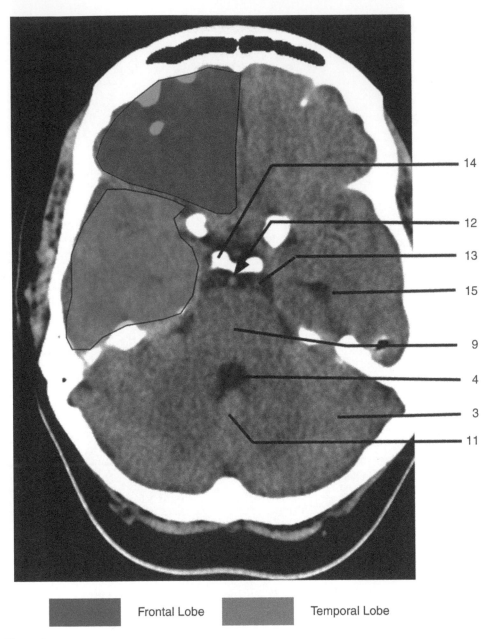

Frontal Lobe   Temporal Lobe

Figure 9

11 = Cerebellar vermis
12 = Basilar artery
13 = Prepontine cistern
14 = Dorsum sellae
15 = Temporal horn of lateral ventricle

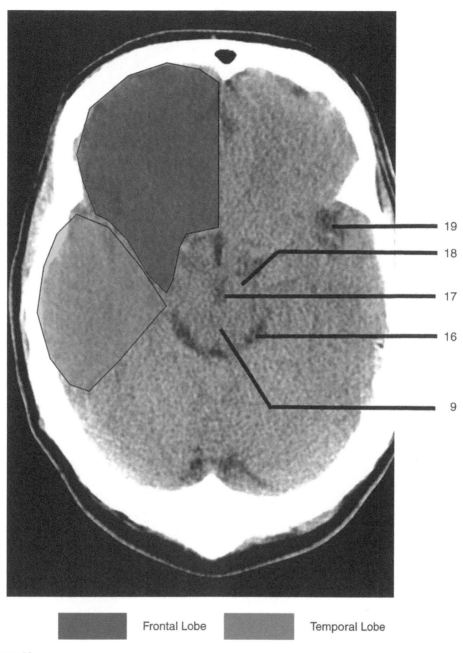

Frontal Lobe   Temporal Lobe

Figure 10

16 = Ambient cistern
17 = Interpeduncular cistern
18 = Cerebral peduncle
19 = Sylvian fissure

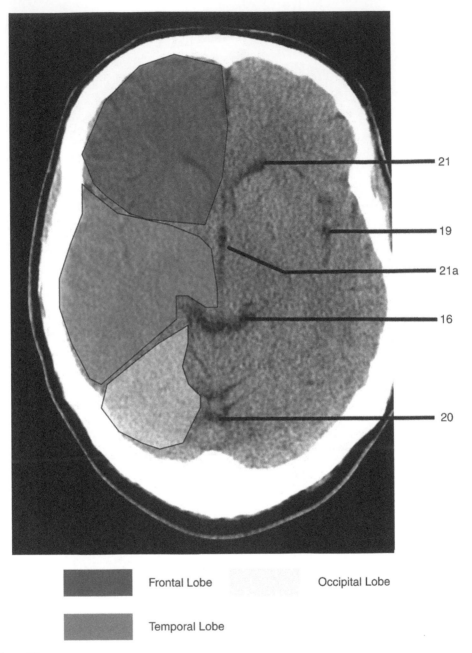

Frontal Lobe   Occipital Lobe

Temporal Lobe

Figure 11

20 = Supra vermian cistern
21 = Frontal horn of lateral ventricle
21a = Third ventricle

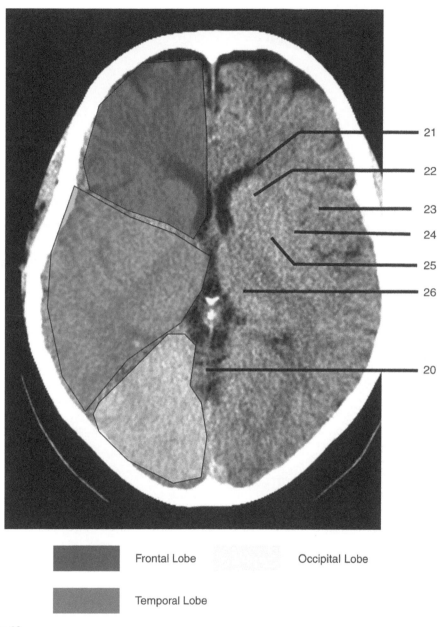

Frontal Lobe   Occipital Lobe

Temporal Lobe

Figure 12

22 = Head of caudate nucleus
23 = Insular cortex
24 = External capsule
25 = Lentiform nucleus
26 = Thalamus

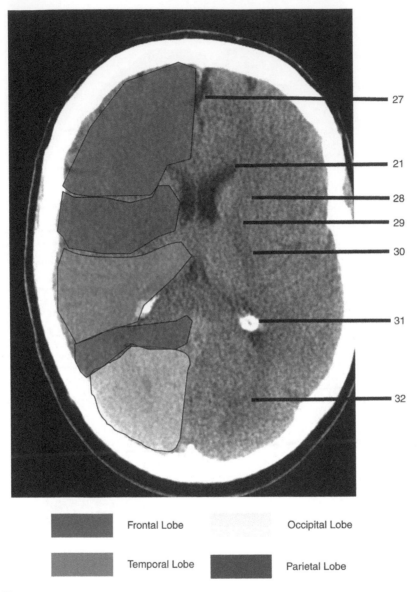

Figure 13

27 = Interhemispheric fissure
28 = Anterior limb of internal capsule
29 = Genu of internal capsule
30 = Posterior limb of internal capsule
31 = Trigone of lateral ventricle and calcified choroid plexus
32 = Occipital horn of lateral ventricle

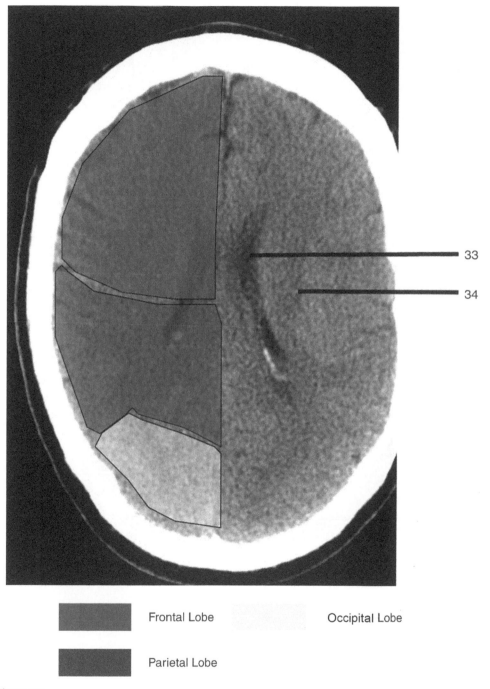

33

34

Frontal Lobe

Occipital Lobe

Parietal Lobe

Figure 14

33 = Body of lateral ventricle
34 = Corona radiata

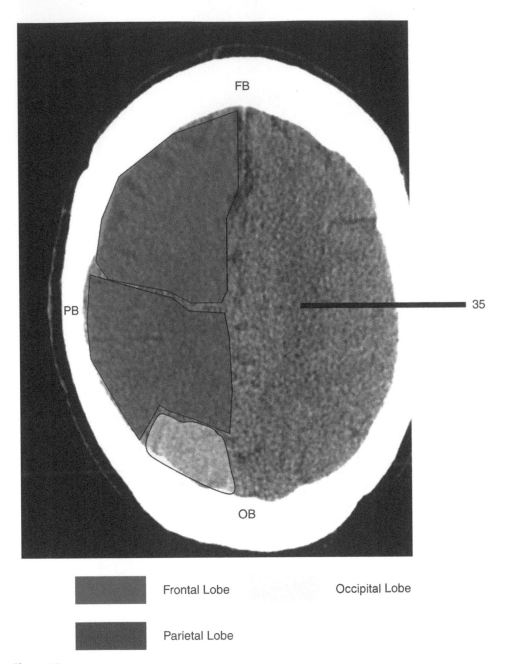

Figure 15

35 = Centrum semiovale
FB = Frontal bone
PB = Parietal bone
OB = Occipital bone

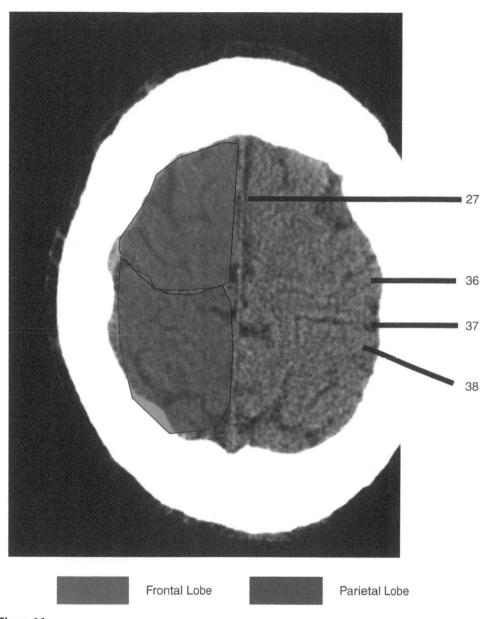

Frontal Lobe   Parietal Lobe

Figure 16

36 = Pre-central gyrus
37 = Central sulcus
38 = Post-central gyrus

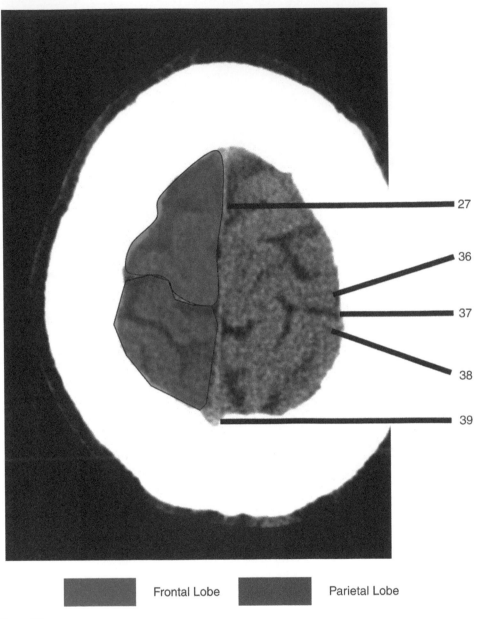

Frontal Lobe   Parietal Lobe

Figure 17

39 = Superior sagittal sinus

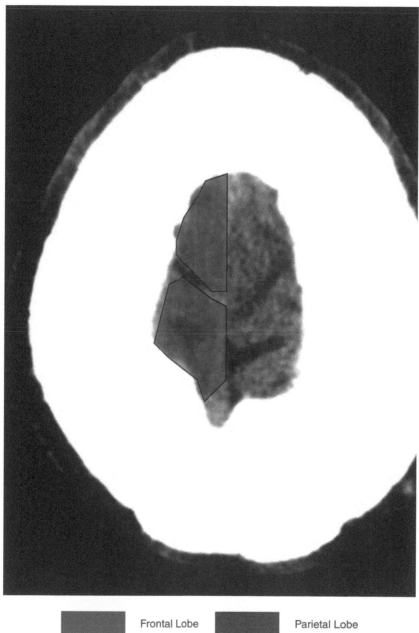

Frontal Lobe   Parietal Lobe

Figure 18

Review of Normal Coronal Anatomy

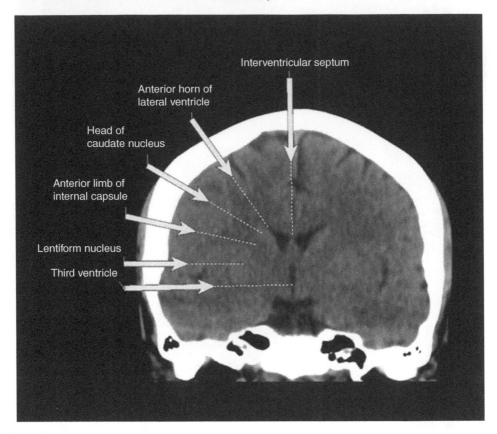

Figure 19

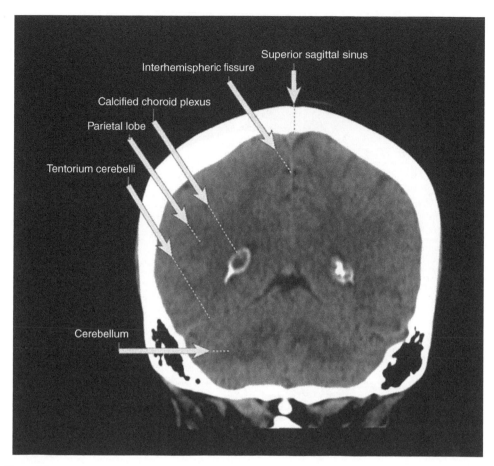

Figure 20

Review of Normal Sagittal Anatomy

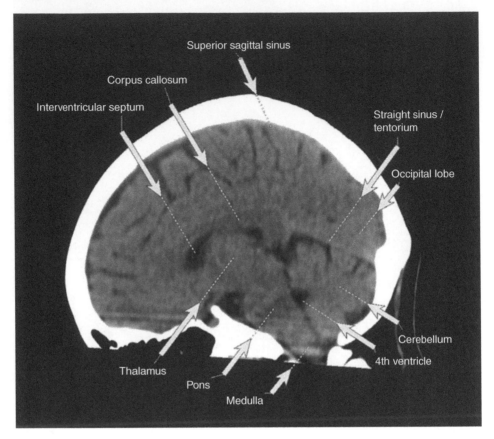

Figure 21

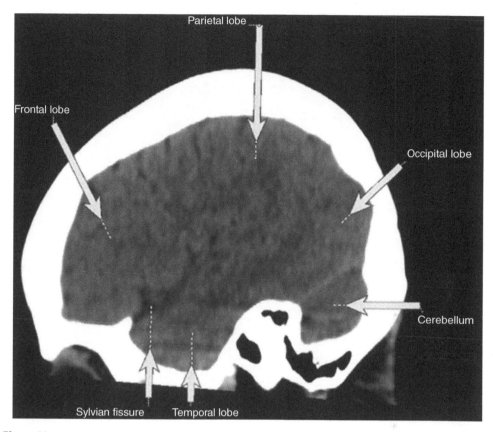

Figure 22

Review of Normal Bony Axial Anatomy

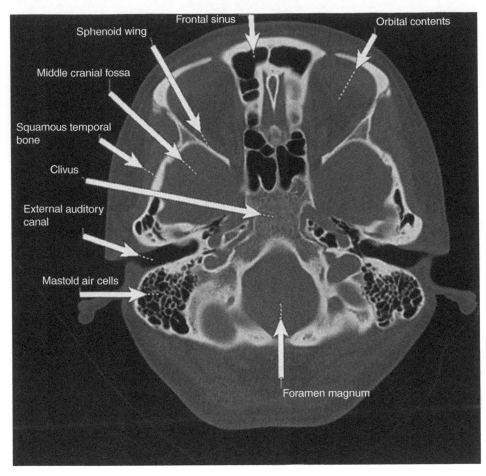

Sphenoid wing
Frontal sinus
Orbital contents
Middle cranial fossa
Squamous temporal bone
Clivus
External auditory canal
Mastold air cells
Foramen magnum

Figure 23

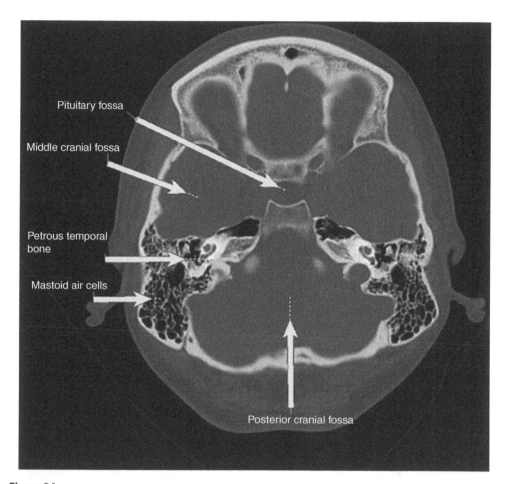

Figure 24

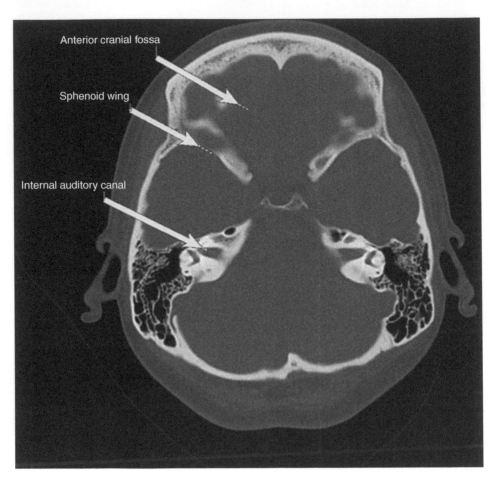

Figure 25

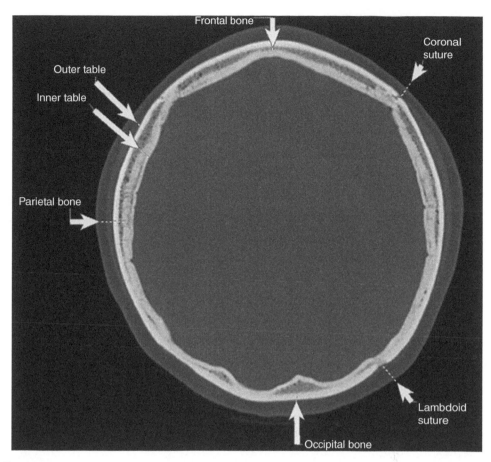

Figure 26

Review of Normal Bony Coronal Anatomy

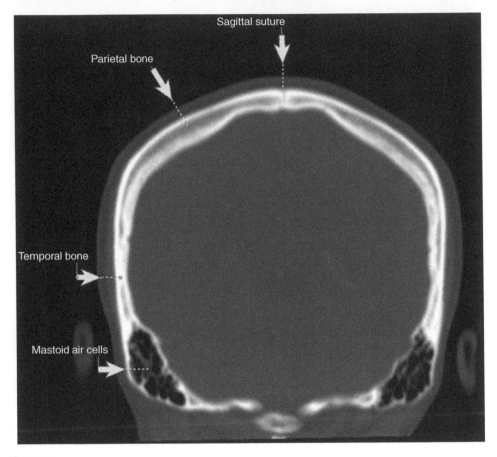

Figure 27

Review of Surface-rendered Bony Anatomy

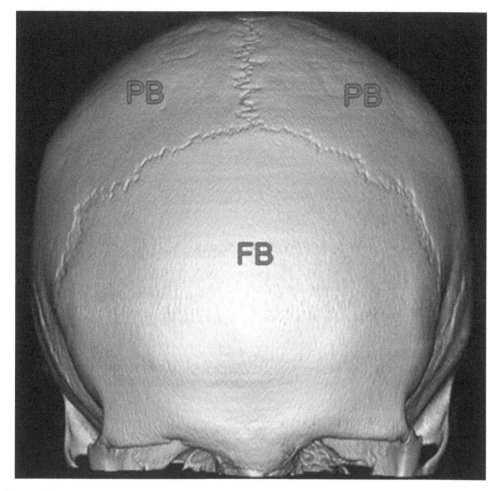

Figure 28

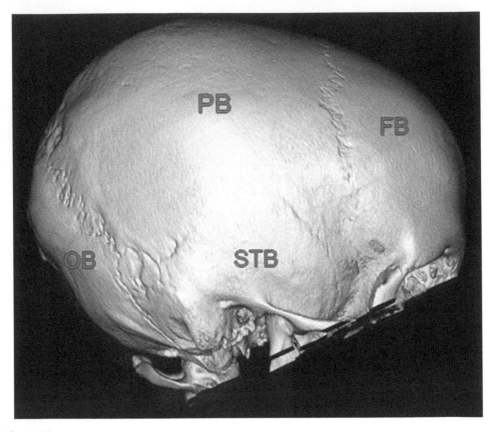

Figure 29

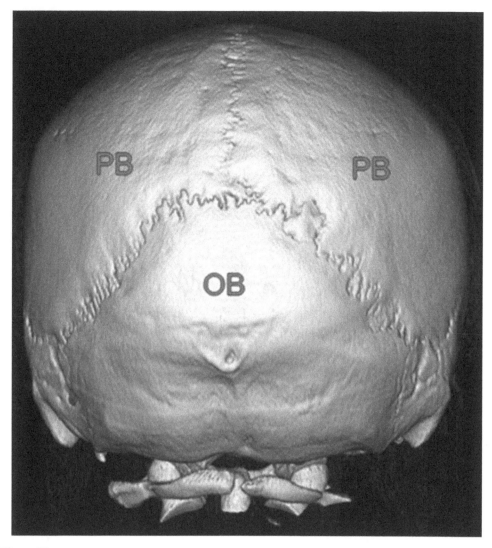

Figure 30

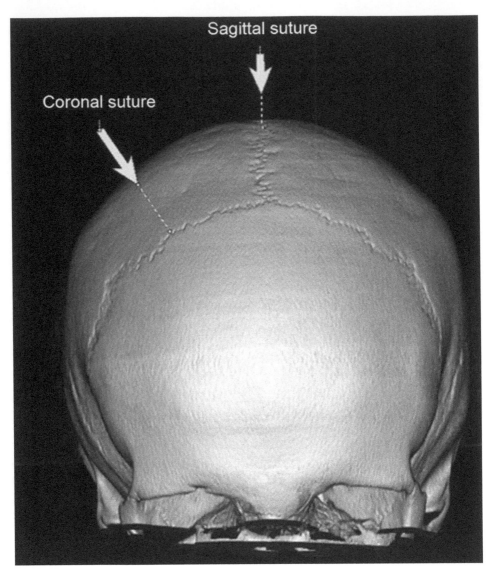

Figure 31

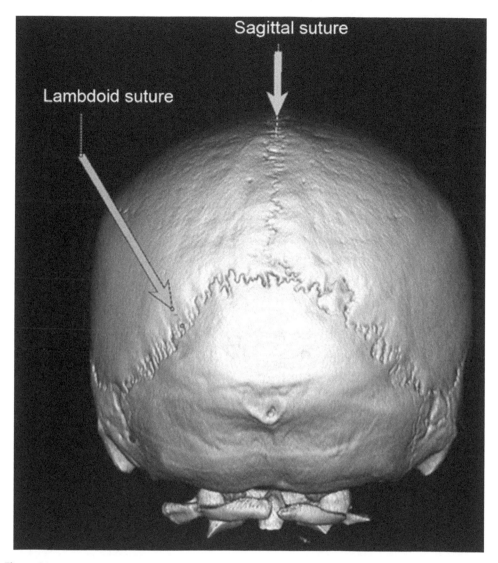

Figure 32

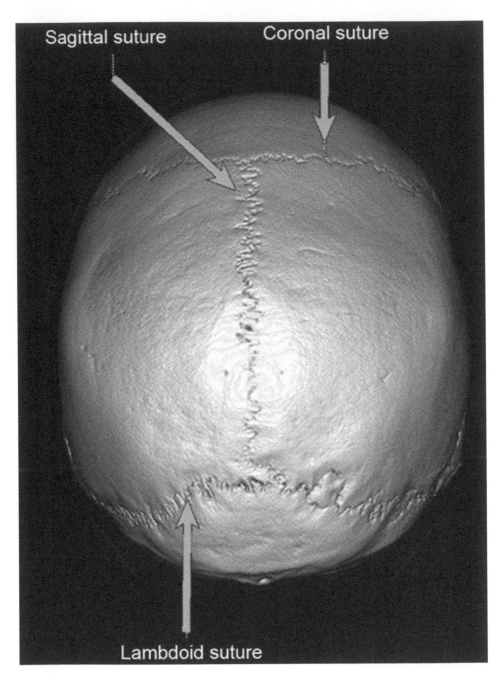

Figure 33

Review of Vascular Territories

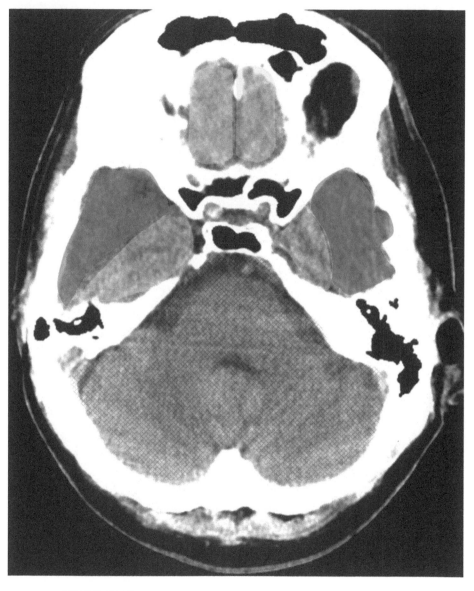

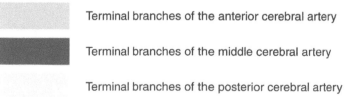

Terminal branches of the anterior cerebral artery

Terminal branches of the middle cerebral artery

Terminal branches of the posterior cerebral artery

Figure 34

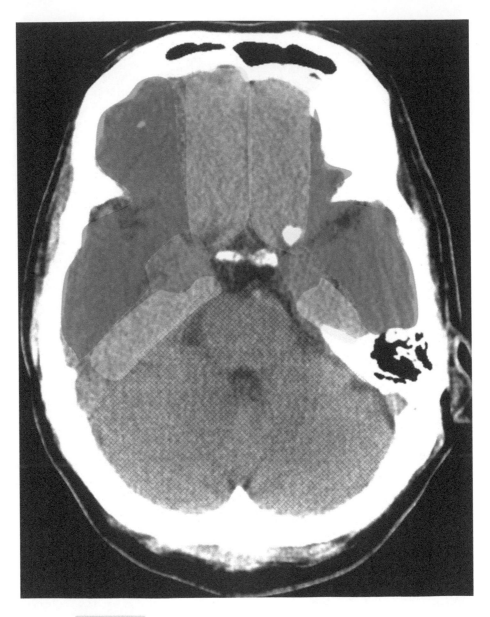

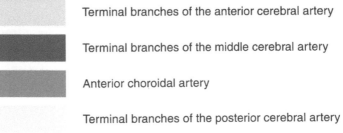

Terminal branches of the anterior cerebral artery

Terminal branches of the middle cerebral artery

Anterior choroidal artery

Terminal branches of the posterior cerebral artery

Figure 35

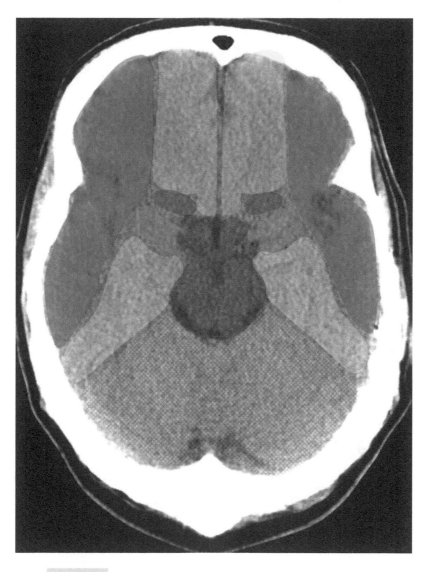

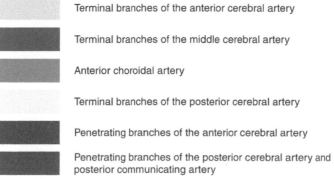

Terminal branches of the anterior cerebral artery

Terminal branches of the middle cerebral artery

Anterior choroidal artery

Terminal branches of the posterior cerebral artery

Penetrating branches of the anterior cerebral artery

Penetrating branches of the posterior cerebral artery and
posterior communicating artery

Figure 36

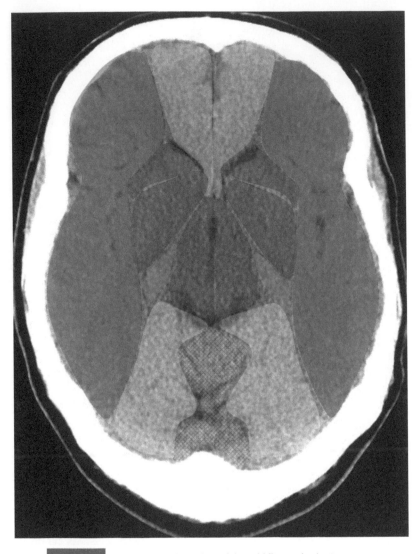

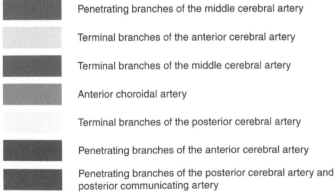

Penetrating branches of the middle cerebral artery

Terminal branches of the anterior cerebral artery

Terminal branches of the middle cerebral artery

Anterior choroidal artery

Terminal branches of the posterior cerebral artery

Penetrating branches of the anterior cerebral artery

Penetrating branches of the posterior cerebral artery and posterior communicating artery

Figure 37

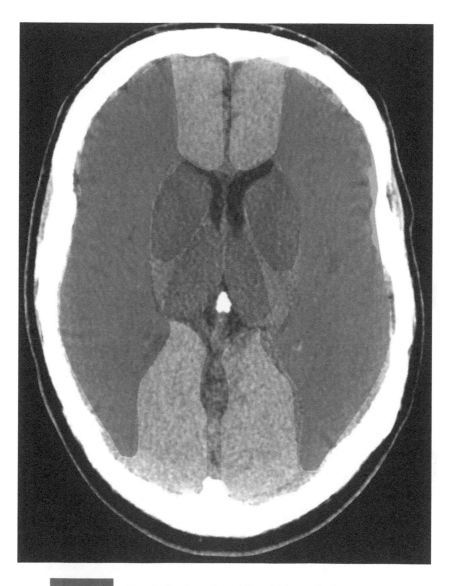

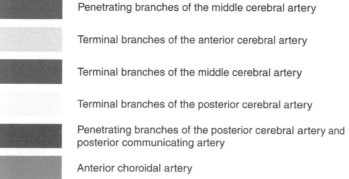

Penetrating branches of the middle cerebral artery

Terminal branches of the anterior cerebral artery

Terminal branches of the middle cerebral artery

Terminal branches of the posterior cerebral artery

Penetrating branches of the posterior cerebral artery and posterior communicating artery

Anterior choroidal artery

Figure 38

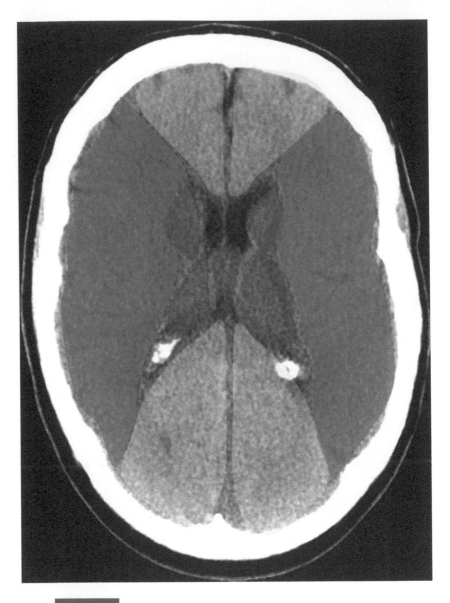

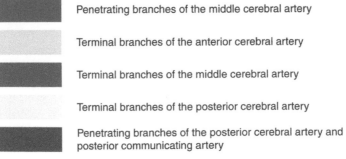

Penetrating branches of the middle cerebral artery

Terminal branches of the anterior cerebral artery

Terminal branches of the middle cerebral artery

Terminal branches of the posterior cerebral artery

Penetrating branches of the posterior cerebral artery and posterior communicating artery

Figure 39

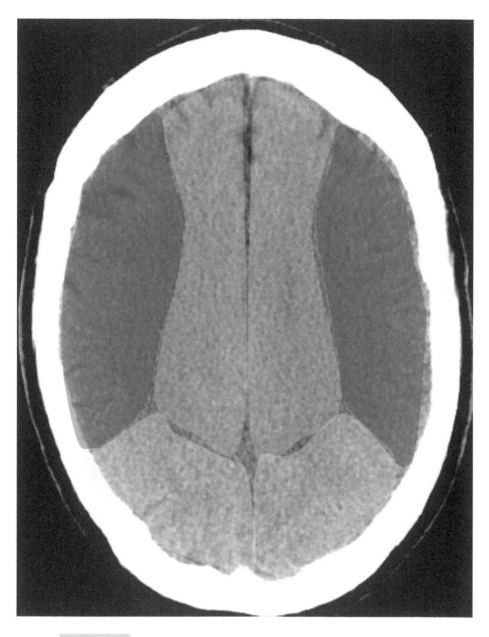

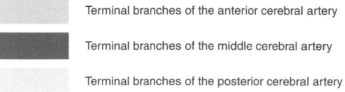

Terminal branches of the anterior cerebral artery

Terminal branches of the middle cerebral artery

Terminal branches of the posterior cerebral artery

Figure 40

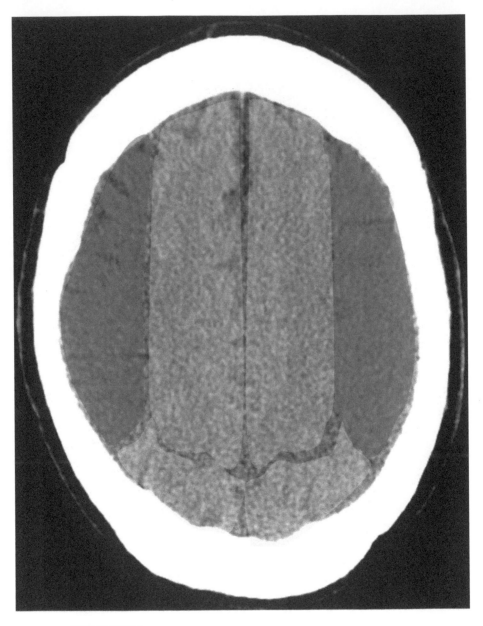

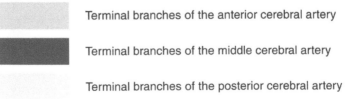

Terminal branches of the anterior cerebral artery

Terminal branches of the middle cerebral artery

Terminal branches of the posterior cerebral artery

Figure 41

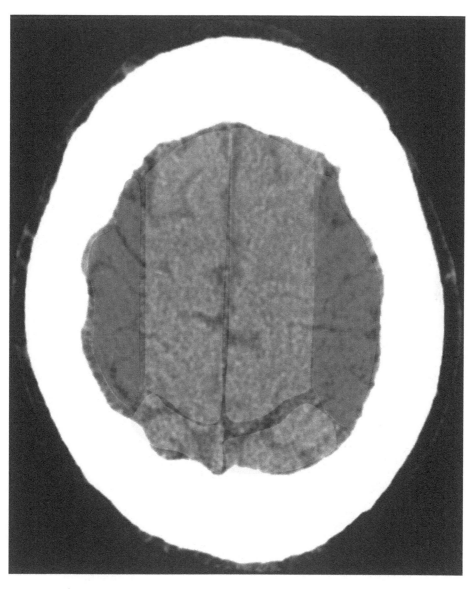

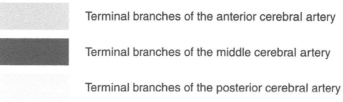

Terminal branches of the anterior cerebral artery

Terminal branches of the middle cerebral artery

Terminal branches of the posterior cerebral artery

Figure 42

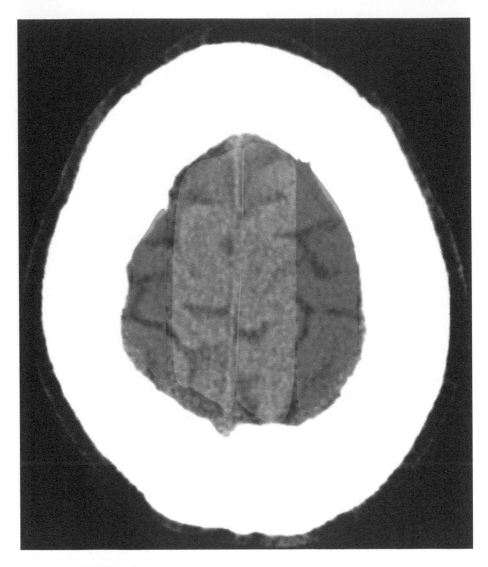

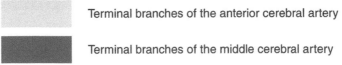

Terminal branches of the anterior cerebral artery

Terminal branches of the middle cerebral artery

Figure 43

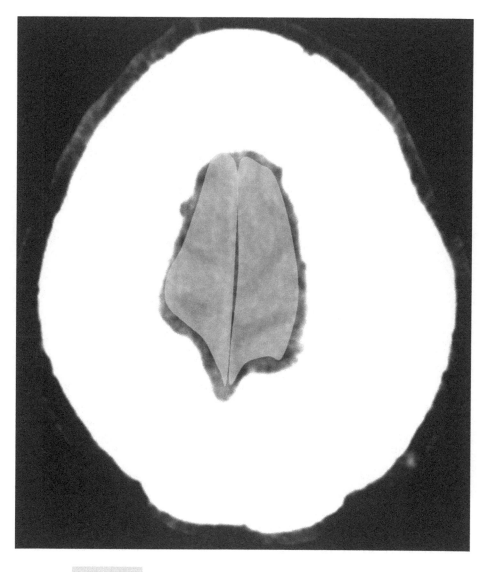

Terminal branches of the anterior cerebral artery

Figure 44

Review of Vascular Anatomy

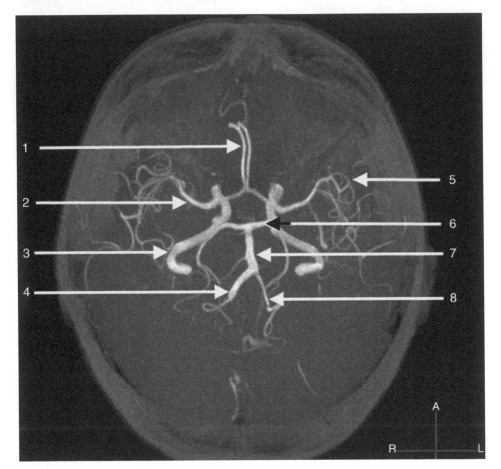

Figure 45

Key for vascular anatomy
1. Anterior cerebral artery
2. Middle cerebral artery
3. Internal carotid artery
4. Right vertebral artery
5. Cortical branches of the middle cerebral artery
6. Posterior cerebral artery
7. Basilar artery
8. Left vertebral artery

Reviewing a CT Scan

Suggested Systematic Approach to Interpretation

- Check patient information and review scan protocol (e.g. non-contrast/contrast-enhanced).
- Check the scout image. May reveal a fracture or gross abnormality not obvious on the axial images. Review alignment of upper cervical vertebrae.
- A quick 'first pass' is recommended, noting gross pathology, followed by a more detailed analysis of the images. Use the mnemonic 'ABBCS' to remember important structures.
- Finally, extend search pattern to include orbits, sinuses, oropharynx, ears, craniocervical junction, face, vault and scalp.

ABBCS

- 'A' – **Asymmetry:** assess all slices, comparing one side to the other, remembering to account for head tilt and to account for various forms of artefact.
- 'B' – **Blood:** acute haemorrhage appears hyperdense in relation to brain, due to clot retraction and water loss. Haemorrhage typically has a CT number in the range of HU_50–100.
  - Assess for both blood overlying the cerebral hemispheres and within the brain parenchyma.
  - Assess the ventricles and CSF spaces for the presence or layering of blood.
  - Review the sulci and fissures for subtle evidence of SAH.
  - Remember slow-flowing blood within a vessel can mimic clot.
  - Conversely, clot within a vessel is an important diagnosis:
    - Venous sinus thrombosis.
    - Dense MCA sign in acute CVA.

- 'B' – **Brain**
  - **Density**
    - Hyperdensity: acute blood (free and within vessels), tumour, bone, contrast and artefact/foreign body.
    - Hypodensity: oedema/infarction, air and tumour.
  - **Displacement**
    - Look for midline shift.
    - Examine midline structures such as the falx cerebri, pituitary and pineal glands.

- Look for asymmetry of CSF spaces such as effacement of an anterior horn of the lateral ventricles or loss of sulcal pattern suggesting oedema.

- **Differentiation of grey/white matter**
  - Normal grey/white matter differentiation should be readily apparent; white matter is of slightly reduced attenuation in comparison to grey matter due to increased fatty myelin content.
  - In an early infarction, oedema leads to loss of the normal grey/white matter differentiation. This can be subtle and again only apparent when comparing both sides; identify normal structures such as internal capsule, thalamus, lentiform and caudate nuclei.

- **'C' – CSF spaces**
  - Assess the sizes of the ventricles and sulci, in proportion to each other and assess the brain parenchyma.
  - Identify normal cisterns (quadrigeminal plate, suprasellar and the mid brain region) and fissures (interhemispheric and Sylvian).
  - The ventricles often hold the key to analysing the image:
    - Pathology may be primary, within a ventricle, or may result from secondary compression from adjacent brain pathology.
    - If a ventricle is enlarged, consider whether it is due to an obstructive/non-communicating or non-obstructive cause. The former depends on site and the latter usually involves pathology in the subarachnoid space.
    - Ex-vacuo dilatation is caused by loss/atrophy of brain tissue, often resulting in abnormal secondary enlargement of the adjacent ventricle. Small ventricles can be normal in children (increase in size with age).
    - Diffuse brain swelling can result in ventricular compression and reduced conspicuity of the normal sulcal/gyral pattern. Causes include metabolic/anoxic injury, infection, trauma and superior sagittal sinus thrombosis.

- **'S' – Skull and scalp**
  - Assess the scalp for soft tissue injury.
  - Can be useful in patients where the full history is absent.
  - Can help to localise coup and contracoup injuries.
  - Carefully assess the bony vault underlying a soft tissue injury for evidence of a fracture.
  - Assess the bony vault for shape, symmetry and mineralisation (focal sclerotic or lytic lesions).
  - Remember to adjust windowing to optimise bony detail.

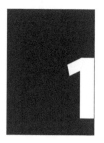

Acute Stroke

Characteristics

- Stroke is the third most common cause of death in the UK. Every year 110,000 people have a stroke in England alone, and stroke is the leading cause of adult disability, with > 300,000 people in England living with moderate to severe disability as a result of stroke.
- Strokes are broadly divided into ischaemic or haemorrhagic. Ischaemic stroke refers to those caused by thrombosis or emboli, and are more common than haemorrhagic stroke.
- Haemorrhagic stroke accounts for 15% of all strokes, usually caused by hypertensive damage to small intracerebral arteries, causing rupture and leakage of blood directly into the parenchyma. This causes surrounding oedema and mass effect, further compromising the adjacent blood supply.
- Transient ischaemic attack (TIA) is defined as a transient episode of neurological dysfunction caused by focal brain, spinal cord, or retinal ischaemia, without acute infarction.
- Many patients who have a TIA will go on to have a stroke. The risk is highest in those patients with carotid artery stenosis or atrial fibrillation. The *ABCD^2 score* (Appendix 1) is widely used in clinical practice to risk-stratify patients for further investigation and treatment.
- The incidence of stroke increases with age, although one-quarter occur in the under 65s.
- Risk factors include hypertension, smoking, diabetes, heart disease (coronary artery disease, cardiomyopathy, chronic atrial fibrillation), hyperlipidaemia, atherosclerosis, the oral contraceptive pill and obesity. Underlying brain pathology (e.g. tumour), bleeding diatheses, anticoagulation treatment and thrombolysis therapy are additional risk factors specific to haemorrhagic strokes. Cocaine use is a risk factor for both ischaemic and haemorrhagic strokes.

Clinical Features

- Haemorrhagic and ischaemic strokes are difficult to distinguish clinically, and the only reliable way to differentiate is with brain imaging. The spectrum of presentation can range from mild symptoms and signs in a well patient, to a moribund comatosed patient.
- Patients with haemorrhagic strokes tend to be more unwell, with abrupt symptom onset and rapid deterioration. Common symptoms include headache, decreased conscious level, seizures, nausea and vomiting. Hypertension is characteristic.

- Ischaemic strokes have a varied presentation depending on the vascular territory involved, commonly presenting with unilateral weakness and/or sensory loss, visual field defect, aphasia and inattention/neglect.
- The neurological deficit can be sudden, often occurring during sleep, making the time of onset difficult to ascertain.
- Posterior circulation strokes commonly present with a varying combination of vertigo, headache, diplopia, ataxia, dysarthria or dysphasia.
- The ROSIER score facilitates recognition of acute stroke (Appendix 2).

Immediate CT Head in a Clinical Stroke

- An immediate CT Head should be performed when the following conditions are met:
  - indications for thrombolysis, or patient is on anticoagulation treatment
  - a known bleeding tendency
  - a depressed level of consciousness (GCS [Glasgow Coma Score] < 13) (Appendix 4)
  - progressive or fluctuating symptoms
  - papilloedema, neck stiffness or fever
  - severe headache at onset of stroke symptoms.

Patients attending with features of acute stroke should be admitted to a dedicated stroke unit to improve long-term.morbidity and mortality (Appendix 3).

Radiological Features

CT

- Aims to identify any contraindication to thrombolysis rather than confirmation of diagnosis.
- Contraindications include:
  - Haemorrhage.
  - >1/3 of MCA territory involvement (increased risk of haemorrhage with thrombolysis and a relative contraindication).
  - Using the 10-point ASPECTS (Alberta Stroke Program Early CT score) system is useful to ensure systematic interpretation of brain CT, and also helps to determine prognosis.

Features

Ischaemic Stroke

Hyperacute infarct (< 12 hours)

- Non-contrast CT may appear normal in up to 60%.
- Contrary to general opinion, the CT may be abnormal in up to 75% of patients with MCA infarction, imaged within the first 3 hours.
- *Hyperdense vessel sign* represents acute intraluminal thrombus, recognised as focal or linear increased (white) density within the artery on non-contrast CT head. This is most commonly seen in MCA occlusion in 25–50% (Fig. 46), although it can be present in other intracranial arteries.

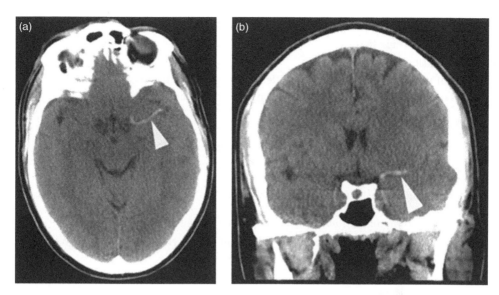

Figure 46 (a) Axial and (b) coronal images demonstrating a hyperdense left MCA in keeping with acute intraluminal thrombus (arrowheads).

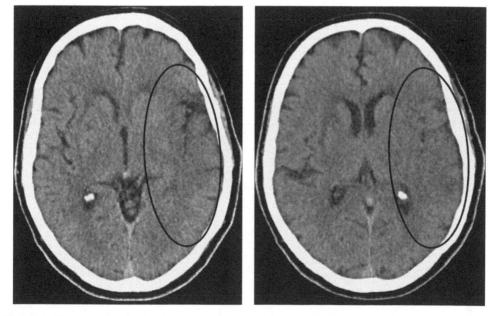

Figure 47 Two examples of early left MCA territory infarction. Note the subtle effacement of grey/white matter differentiation, due to oedema, and the 'insular ribbon sign'.

- *Lentiform sign* denotes obscuration of the normally well-defined lentiform nucleus, occurring in 50–80% of acute MCA occlusions.
- *Insular ribbon sign* describes the loss of grey/white matter differentiation in the lateral margins of the insular cortex, supplied by the insular segment of the MCA (Fig. 47).

Acute infarction
12–24 hours (Fig. 48a)

- Low-density basal ganglia.
- Loss of normal grey/white matter differentiation secondary to oedema.
- Loss of the normal sulcal pattern is suspicious of underlying oedema.

1–7 days (Fig. 48b)

- Area of hypodensity in a vascular distribution (in 70% of cases) due to cytotoxic oedema.
- Mass effect secondary to oedema resulting in local or generalised compression of the ventricles, basal cisterns and midline shift.
- Haemorrhagic transformation may occur after 2–4 days in up to 70% of patients.

Subacute/chronic infarction (> 7 days–months) (Fig. 49 and Fig. 50)

- Decrease in mass effect and ex-vacuo dilatation of the ventricles to occupy the potential space resulting from infarcted brain parenchyma.
- Loss of parenchymal mass, with associated sulcal/ventricular widening, due to encephalomalacia.

Haemorrhagic Stroke

- Non-contrast head CT is the investigation of choice as contrast may obscure haematoma, which also appears dense on CT.
- Acute haemorrhage is hyperdense (Fig. 51 and Fig. 52).
- Surrounding oedema will result in loss of the grey/white matter differentiation.

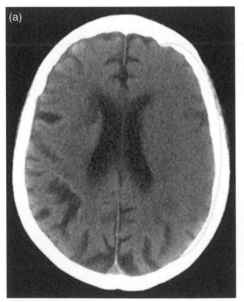 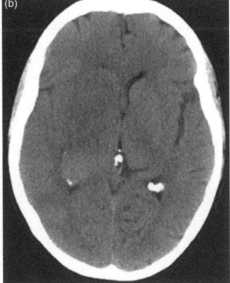

Figure 48 (a) Early large left MCA infarct: axial image showing loss of grey/white matter differentiation and sulcal effacement secondary to oedema in the left MCA territory. (b) Early large right MCA infarct: obscuration of the right lentiform nucleus with low-attenuation oedema causing mass effect, compressing the right lateral ventricle.

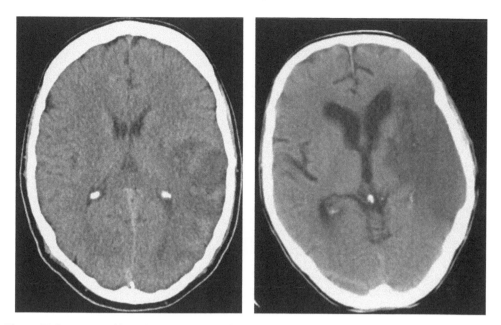

Figure 49 Large areas of hypodensity within the left MCA territory due to cytotoxic oedema.

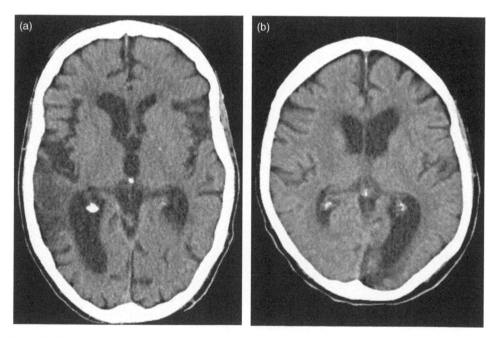

Figure 50 Chronic (a) right MCA and (b) left PCA territory infarcts, demonstrating encephalomalacia (CSF filling the 'dead' space following infarction) and ex-vacuo dilatation of the adjacent ventricle.

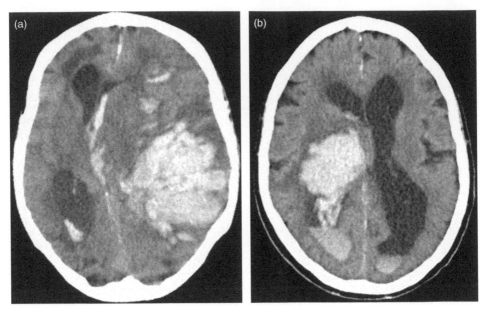

Figure 51 (a) Large intracerebral haemorrhage within the left MCA territory, with rupture into the ventricular system. There is significant mass effect, with shift of midline structures to the right, and compression of the ipsilateral ventricle. (b) Acute haemorrhage centred on the right thalamus and lentiform nucleus with intraventricular rupture.

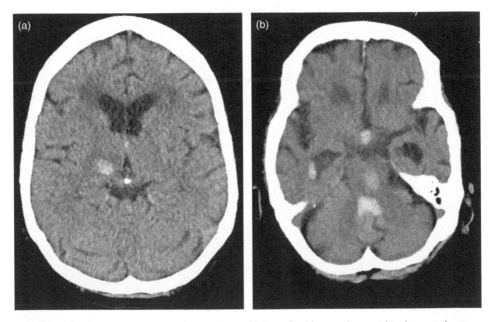

Figure 52 (a) Small acute right thalamic haemorrhage. (b) Acute focal haemorrhage within the central pons. Additional acute intraventricular haemorrhage.

- Mass effect will result in compression of overlying sulci, ventricular compression, midline shift and reduction in the size of the basal cisterns.
- Site and size of the haemorrhage are important, and will influence future treatment options.

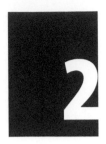

Subdural Haematoma (SDH)

Characteristics

- Subdural haemorrhage arises between the dura and arachnoid membrane of the brain.
- Bleeding results from torn bridging veins that cross the potential space between the cerebral cortex and dural venous sinuses.
- Usually categorised into acute, subacute or chronic.
- Acute subdural haematoma (SDH) carries a high risk of mortality and morbidity, as it is more commonly associated with extensive primary brain injury. Direct pressure results in ischaemia on the adjacent brain tissue.
- Rebleeding secondary to osmotic expansion, or further trauma, leads to acute-on-chronic haemorrhage.
- All causes of brain tissue loss (e.g. hydrocephalus and stroke) are considered risk factors. Elderly and alcohol-dependent patients' risks are often compounded by instability of gait and comorbidity.
- The aetiology of chronic SDH is often unclear, although most likely from minor trauma in the preceding few weeks. In 50% of cases, no such history is obtainable.
- Subdural haemorrhage in the newborn is usually due to obstetric trauma. In paediatric patients, non-accidental injury needs to be considered.

Clinical Features

Acute SDH

- Patients often present following severe head trauma, 50% associated with underlying brain injury, with a worse long-term prognosis than extradural haematoma.
- Patients generally have a decreased level of consciousness, with focal neurological defects or seizures. There may be signs of raised intracranial pressure.
- Patients with a primary or secondary coagulopathy (e.g. alcoholics, those undergoing anticoagulation therapy) may develop an acute SDH after only minor head trauma.
- A small acute SDH may be asymptomatic.

Chronic SDH

- Chronic SDH is the result of:
  - Resolving phase of medically managed acute subdural haematoma.
  - Repeated episodes of subclinical haemorrhage, later becoming symptomatic.

- Chronic SDH often presents in the elderly with vague symptoms of gradual depression, personality change, fluctuation of consciousness, unexplained headaches, or evolving hemiplegia. Over 75% of cases occur in patients > 50 years of age.

Radiological Features

CT

- CT scan without contrast, as high-density contrast may obscure visualisation of blood.

Location

- Blood is seen over the cerebral convexity, often extending into the interhemispheric fissure, along the tentorial margins, and beneath the temporal and occipital lobes (Fig. 53).
- Does not cross the midline, as it is limited by the falx cerebri.
- Bilateral in 15–25% of adults (most commonly in the elderly) and in 80–85% of infants.

Features

Acute SDH (< 72 hours) (Fig. 54)

- Peripheral high-density crescentic fluid collection between the skull and cerebral hemisphere usually with:

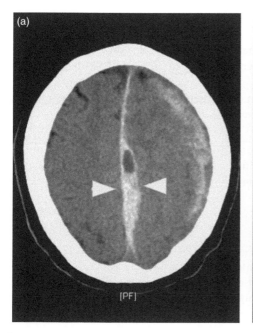
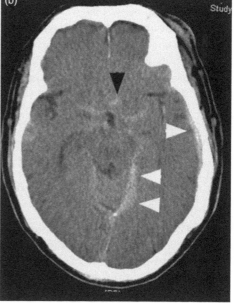

Figure 53 Acute subdural haematoma on axial images (a) over the left cerebral convexity with additional acute-on-chronic haematoma extending along the interhemispheric fissure (arrowheads); (b) along the tentorium and over the left temporal lobe (white arrowheads). Additional subarachnoid haemorrhage is also present (black arrowhead).

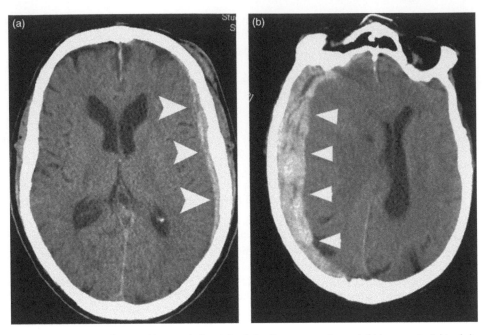

Figure 54 Axial images showing (a) acute shallow left subdural haematoma (arrows); (b) large acute right subdural haematoma (arrowheads).

- A concave inner margin: a small haematoma may only minimally displace brain substance.
- Convex outer margin following normal contour of cranial vault.
- Occasionally, a blood-fluid level is seen secondary to high- and low-density fluid separation.
- Signs of mass effect with compression of overlying sulci, ventricular compression, midline shift and reduction in the size of the basal cisterns.

Subacute SDH (3–21 days) (Fig. 55)

- After approximately 1–2 weeks, the subdural collection becomes isodense to grey matter. Detection may be challenging and may only be recognised due to persistent mass effect:
  - Effacement of cortical sulci.
  - Deviation of lateral ventricle.
  - Midline shift, white-matter buckling.
  - Displacement of grey–white matter interfaces.
- On contrast-enhanced CT scans, the cortical–subdural interface will be defined, with enhancement of the cerebral cortex and non-enhancement of the overlying haematoma.

Chronic SDH (> 21 days) (Fig. 56)

- These are often hypodense crescentic collections, with or without mass effect.

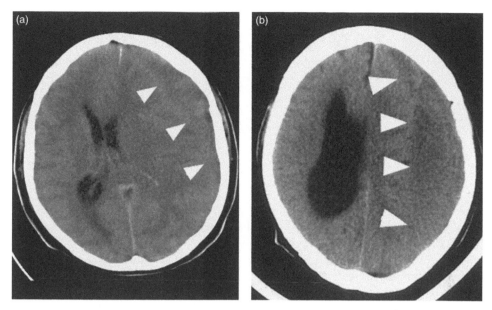

Figure 55 Axial images showing (a) left isodense/hypodense subdural collection (arrowheads) with midline shift to the right; (b) large isodense subdural haematoma (arrowheads) with associated mass effect, compressing the left lateral ventricle and dilatation of the right lateral ventricle.

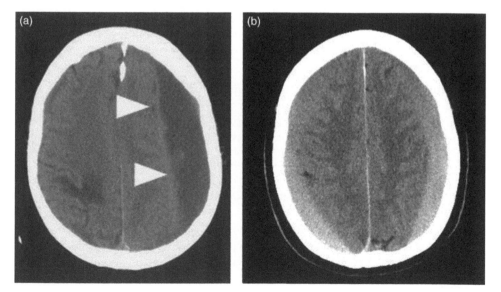

Figure 56 Axial images showing (a) large left chronic subdural haematoma (arrowheads); (b) bilateral chronic subdural haematomas.

- Acute-on-chronic SDHs can further complicate the imaging, with hyperdense fresh haemorrhage intermixed, or layering posteriorly, within the chronic collection.
- Complex septated collections, and in rare cases calcification, may develop.

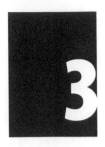

3

Extradural/Epidural Haematoma

Characteristics

- Extra-axial haemorrhage arising within the potential space between the skull and dura mater.
- The dura becomes more adherent with age. The young are more frequently affected, as the dura is more easily stripped away from the skull.
- Associated with a skull fracture in 75–95% of cases.
- Occurs in 2% of all serious head injuries, although seen in < 1% of all children with cranial trauma, as calvarial plasticity means that skull fractures are less common. In rare cases, extradural haematomas can occur spontaneously.
- Bleeding is commonly from a lacerated (middle) meningeal artery/vein, adjacent to the inner skull table, from a fracture crossing the path of the artery or dural branches.
- Early diagnosis is imperative, as prognosis is good with early intervention prior to neurological deterioration from cerebral herniation and brainstem compression.
- Types:
  - Acute extradural haematoma (60%) from arterial bleeding.
  - Subacute extradural haematoma (30%).
  - Chronic extradural haematoma (10%) from venous bleeding or a torn dural sinus (more common with posterior skull fractures).

Clinical Features

- Patients often present with a history of head trauma associated with a variable level of consciousness.
- The classical 'talk and die' presentation, where a brief loss of consciousness occurs at the time of impact, followed by rapid neurological deterioration as the haematoma expands, only occurs in 20–50% of patients. Other symptoms may include headache, vomiting and seizures following head injury.
- Neurological examination may reveal lateralising signs, with a unilateral up-going plantar reflex.
- A sensitive sign in the conscious patient is pronator drift of the upper limb.
- Close neurological observation is necessary to detect any alteration in consciousness, with changes in *Glasgow coma scale* (GCS) (see Appendix 3) and rising intracranial pressure; clinically manifest as dilated, sluggish or fixed pupils, decerebrate posture or Cushing response (hypertension, bradycardia and bradypnoea).

Radiological Features

CT

- CT scan without contrast, as high-density contrast may obscure visualisation of blood.

Location

- 66% temporoparietal (most often from laceration of the middle meningeal artery).
- 29% frontal pole, parieto-occipital region, between occipital lobes and posterior fossa (most often from laceration of the dural sinuses from a fracture).
- Disruption of the sagittal sinus may create a vertex epidural haematoma.

Features

- Biconvex, hyperdense elliptical collection with a sharply defined edge (Fig. 57).
- Mixed high and low density suggests active bleeding, giving a 'whorled' appearance to the haematoma.
- Haematoma does not cross suture lines unless a diastatic suture fracture is present.
- Crosses dural reflections. May separate the venous sinuses and falx from the skull; this is the only type of intracranial haemorrhage to do this.
- Signs of mass effect such as sulcal effacement, ventricular compression, subfalcine herniation, effacement of the basal cisterns and tonsillar herniation may be present.
- Venous bleeding is more variable in shape.
- The study should be carefully scrutinised on bone windows due to the frequent association of skull fractures and extradural haematomas.

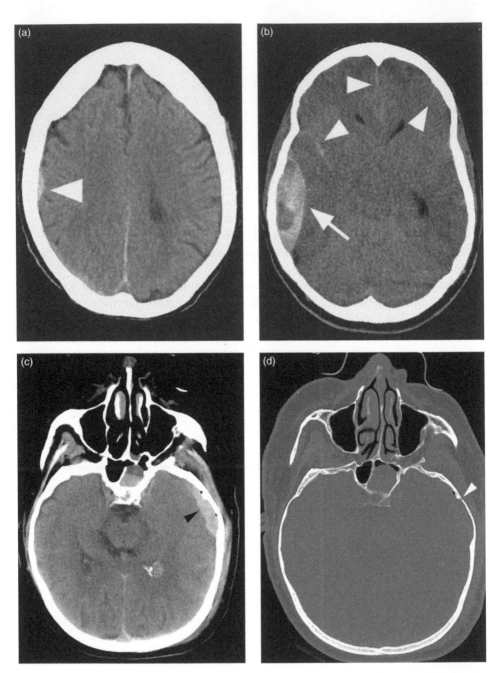

Figure 57 Axial images demonstrating (a) subtle right acute extradural haemorrhage (arrowhead); (b) mixed-density right extradural haemorrhage indicating acute and subacute components (arrow). Note additional subarachnoid haemorrhage (arrowheads); (c) left extradural haemorrhage (black arrowhead) with low-attenuation gas locules secondary to an underlying skull fracture identified on (d) bone windows (white arrowhead). There is also high-attenuation blood within the left sphenoid sinus.

Subarachnoid Haemorrhage

Characteristics

- Subarachnoid haemorrhage (SAH) accounts for 6–8% of cerebrovascular accidents (CVAs). Recognised as a particularly important cause in younger patients. Its incidence remains constant despite other causes of CVAs showing a decrease.
- Causes:
  - Spontaneous – ruptured aneurysm (72%), arteriovenous malformation (AVM) (10%) and hypertensive haemorrhage.
  - Trauma.
- Blood enters the subarachnoid space between the pia and arachnoid mater which may lead to raised intracranial pressure by obstructing the ventricular outflow of CSF.
- Incidence increases with age and peaks at age 50 years. Approximately 80% of cases of SAH occur in people aged 40–65 years, with 15% occurring in people aged 20–40 years.
- 40–50% of patients with aneurysmal SAH have symptoms from a 'sentinel bleed' consistent with a small leak. This may occur a few hours to a few months before the rupture, with a median time of 2 weeks prior to diagnosis.
- An estimated 10–15% of patients die before reaching hospital and the mortality rate approaches 40% within the first week due to rebleeding.
- Advances in management have resulted in reduced mortality, although more than one-third of survivors have major residual neurological deficits leading to long-term morbidity.

Clinical Features

- SAH classically presents with a sudden onset of a severe 'thunderclap' headache, often described as the 'worst headache in my life'.
- Meningeal irritation generates symptoms of neck stiffness, photophobia and low back pain, with a positive Kernig's sign.
- 10–25% of patients develop seizures within minutes of the onset.
- Rise in intracranial pressure can lead to nausea and vomiting.
- Prodromal symptoms may also be reported and are not necessarily related to a 'sentinel bleed'.
- Focal neurological signs:
  - Oculomotor nerve palsy – compression by an expanding berry aneurysm of the posterior communicating artery of the circle of Willis.

- Abducens nerve palsy – associated with increased intracranial pressure.
- Mono-ocular visual loss due to ophthalmic artery aneurysm.
- Unilateral leg weakness or paraparesis suggests anterior communicating artery aneurysm rupture.

- Fundoscopy may reveal papilloedema and subhyaloid retinal haemorrhages.
- Lumbar puncture (LP) is performed 12 hours after the onset of symptoms to evaluate for xanthochromia if the initial CT is negative for SAH. 15% of LPs are false negatives.

Radiological Features

CT

- CT scan without contrast, as high-density contrast may obscure visualisation of blood.

Location of Aneurysm Rupture

- Approximately 85% of saccular aneurysms occur in the anterior circulation. The most common sites of rupture are as follows:
  - The internal carotid artery, including the posterior communicating (PCom) artery junction (41%).
  - The anterior communicating (ACom) artery/anterior cerebral artery (34%).
  - The middle cerebral artery (MCA) (20%).
  - The vertebrobasilar and other arteries (5%).

Features

- CT scan findings are positive in approximately 92% of patients who have SAH.
- Sensitivity decreases with time; 98% within the first 12 hours and 93% within 24 hours. This decreases to 80% at 72 hours and 50% at 1 week.
- May be falsely negative in patients with small haemorrhages and in those with severe anaemia.
- The aneurysm may be apparent as a round soft-tissue density structure with or without rim calcification (Fig. 58).
- The location of blood within the subarachnoid space correlates directly with the location of the aneurysm rupture in 70% of cases:
  - Internal carotid artery – 4th ventricle, basal cistern and around brainstem.
  - ACom artery – interhemispheric and frontal horn intraventricular blood (Fig. 59a).
  - MCA – Sylvian fissure and temporal lobe haematoma (Fig. 60a).
  - Vertebrobasilar arteries – interpeduncular or cerebellopontine angle cistern (Fig. 59b).
  - Blood found lying over the cerebral convexities or within the superficial brain parenchyma suggests rupture of an AVM or mycotic aneurysm.
- Mass effect: hydrocephalus and subfalcine/transtentorial herniation. This is due to reduced outflow/resorption of CSF by arachnoid granulations secondary to the haemorrhage, and may be present in up to 20% of patients.

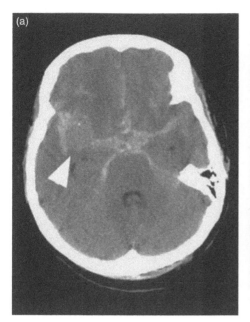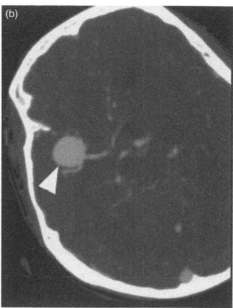

Figure 58 (a) Axial image demonstrating extensive hyperdense subarachnoid blood within the basal cisterns secondary to a ruptured right MCA aneurysm (arrowhead); (b) CT angiogram showing large right MCA aneurysm (arrowhead).

- Subtle areas for review: high density within sulci, occipital horn of the lateral ventricles (blood/fluid level), interpeduncular cistern, and asymmetrical density of the tentorium cerebelli (Fig. 61, Fig. 62).
- A contrast-enhanced CT scan may reveal an underlying AVM; however, a non-contrast study should always be performed first.

CT Angiography

Features

- There is continuing debate regarding its sensitivity compared with the gold standard of catheter angiography. It has the advantage of being non-invasive, reducing the small but important neurological risks related to conventional catheter angiography.
- Recent meta-analysis shows a sensitivity of 57–100% compared with conventional angiography and surgical findings, with higher sensitivity observed with newer multi-slice scanners. The most commonly missed aneurysms are those < 4 mm in size and adjacent to the skull base.
- Uses a combination of multiplanar reformat, maximal intensity projection (Fig. 60b) and volume and surface rendering from the source images. This allows identification and depiction of aneurysm anatomy including: aneurysm location, size, neck, orientation, and relationship to parent vessel, adjacent vessels and other structures. The anatomy will determine patient management with endovascular coiling or surgical clipping.
- Best performed by experienced radiologists using protocols agreed with a neurosurgical centre.

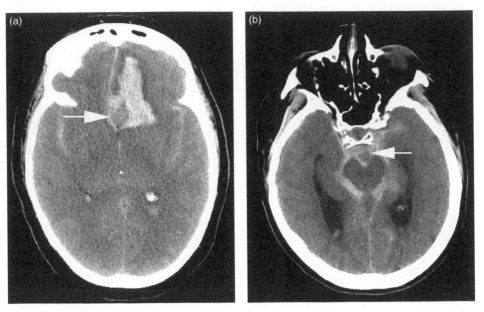

Figure 59 (a) Axial image demonstrating extensive hyperdense blood in the left frontal lobe, interhemispheric fissure, Sylvian fissures bilaterally and occipital horn, secondary to rupture of an anterior communication artery aneurysm (arrow). (b) Axial image demonstrating extensive hyperdense blood within the interpeduncular and ambient cisterns secondary to rupture of a basilar artery tip aneurysm (arrow).

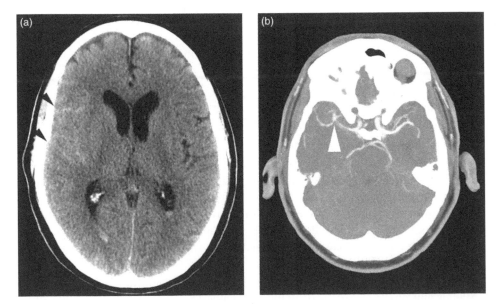

Figure 60 (a) Axial image demonstrating subtle hyperdense subarachnoid blood within the right convexity sulci (black arrowheads). There is layering of blood in the occipital horns of the lateral ventricles. (b) Maximum-intensity projection image from a CT angiogram showing small right MCA aneurysm (arrowhead).

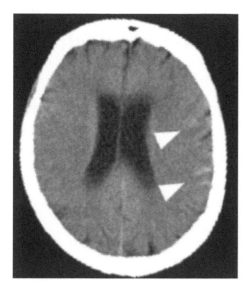

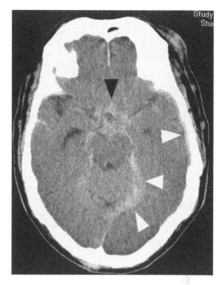

Figure 61 An example of subtle subarachnoid haemorrhage. Faint hyperdense subarachnoid blood is seen outlining cerebral sulci (arrowheads).

Figure 62 Subarachnoid blood within the suprasellar cistern (black arrowhead). Additional acute subdural haemorrhage along the tentorium and over the left temporal lobe (white arrowheads).

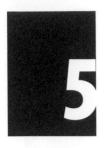

Traumatic Parenchymal Brain Injury

5

Characteristics of Head Injury

- Head injuries account for about 1.5 million attendances each year to emergency departments.
- Traumatic brain injury usually results from linear acceleration/deceleration forces or penetrating injuries.
- Incidence of head injury is difficult to assess, as patients with mild injury do not present, while those with severe injury often die at the scene of the incident and are therefore under-reported.
- Fatal outcomes are more likely in those whose presenting GCS is < 8.
- Can be subcategorised into: primary injury, including contusion and diffuse axonal injury; and secondary injury, including diffuse cerebral oedema and brain herniation.

Clinical Features

- Usually a history of head trauma or external signs of injury.
- Altered or fluctuating GCS.
- Headache +/− vomiting.
- Pupil asymmetry.
- Otorrhoea/rhinorrhoea/Battle's sign/raccoon eyes may be present in basal skull fracture.
- Focal neurological deficit may occur if contusions arise near the sensorimotor cortex.
- Most patients make an uneventful recovery, but a few develop raised intracranial pressure, post-traumatic seizures and persisting focal neurological deficits.
- Lower threshold for scanning in the presence of anticoagulant therapy.
- CT scan indications – see Appendix 5 and Appendix 7.

Radiological Features

CT

- CT scan without contrast as high-density contrast may obscure visualisation of blood.

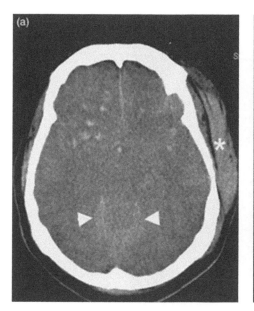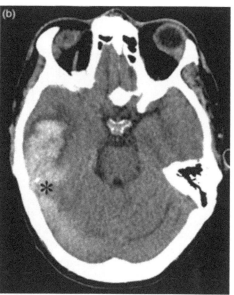

Figure 63 Axial images demonstrating (a) multifocal contusions within both frontal lobes, with additional acute subarachnoid haemorrhage along the basal cisterns and tentorium (arrowheads), marked frontoparietal soft-tissue swelling (asterisk); (b) large right temporal contusion (asterisk).

Features

Contusion

- Solitary or multiple foci of high-density hematomas in the cortical or subcortical region, representing primary parenchymal and vascular injuries (Fig. 63).
- Most commonly located in the anterior, lateral and inferior surfaces of the frontal and temporal lobes; thought to be related to the relative irregularity of the skull base at these sites.
- Parenchymal injury adjacent to site of external trauma is termed '*Coup injury*'. A '*Contra coup*' injury results from the impact of the moving brain against the inner skull table, opposite to the site of direct injury. Paradoxically often larger than the 'Coup injury'.
- The resulting cell damage leads to cytotoxic brain oedema, resulting in regional ischaemia, appearing as hypodense areas of brain parenchyma in association with the high-density contusion.

Diffuse Axonal Injury

- Small and multiple lesions of high attenuation secondary to widespread disruption of axons during acceleration/deceleration injury.
- Typically located in the corpus callosal complex, parasagittal grey/white matter junction, deep periventricular white matter (especially in the frontal areas), basal ganglia, internal capsule, hippocampal and parahippocampal regions, brain stem and cerebellum (Fig. 64).

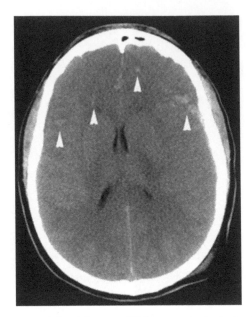

Figure 64 Axial image showing multiple subtle areas of high attenuation in the frontal lobes bilaterally (arrowheads) at grey–white matter junctions and deep white matter, in keeping with diffuse axonal injury.

- Focal haematomas and diffuse axonal injury are more accurately assessed on MR imaging than CT. A gradient recall echo sequence is recommended for its ability to detect susceptibility artefact from haemosiderin secondary to haemorrhage. However, this is infrequently used in the acute setting due to length of examination and safety of patient transfer.

Diffuse Cerebral Oedema

- Results from either hyperaemia or interstitial oedema. Leads to effacement of sulci, loss of the suprasellar and quadrigeminal cisterns and compression of the ventricles.
- Generalised homogeneous low-attenuation parenchyma represents diffuse loss of grey/white matter differentiation secondary to oedema. The cerebellum may appear hyperdense in comparison – *'white cerebellum'* sign (Fig. 65a).
- The diffuse low density of the cerebrum can produce a *'Pseudo-subarachnoid haemorrhage'* appearance as the dura and vessels appear relatively hyperdense against the brain parenchyma (Fig. 65b).

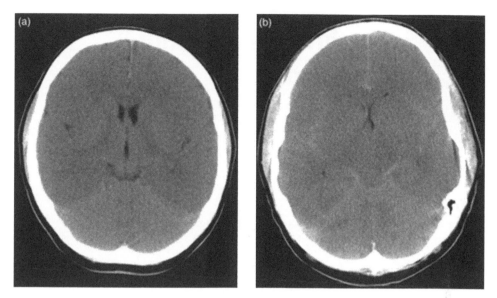

Figure 65 Axial images showing diffuse low-attenuation cerebral parenchyma causing (a) relative hyperdensity of the cerebellum – white cerebellum sign; (b) relative hyperdensity of the blood vessels and meninges and effacement of the basal cisterns – pseudo-subarachnoid haemorrhage appearance.

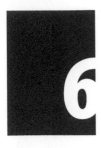

Cerebral Venous Sinus Thrombosis

6

Characteristics
- Rare cause of stroke, more common in younger age groups with a female preponderance.
- Risk factors:
    - *Septic causes (esp. in childhood):*

      Intracranial infections: meningitis, encephalitis, brain abscess, empyema.
      Locoregional infection: mastoiditis.

    - *Aseptic causes:*

      Hypercoagulable states: polycythaemia rubra vera, idiopathic thrombocytosis, thrombocytopaenia.
      Hormonal: pregnancy, oral contraceptive pill.

    - *Trauma:*

      Head injury.
      Iatrogenic procedures: lumbar puncture, neurosurgical intervention.

    - *Low-flow state:*

      Dehydration, CCF, shock.

    - In approximately 1/3 of patients, no cause is found.

Clinical Features
- Sudden-onset severe headache (75%) – may mimic SAH.
- Focal neurological deficit (50%).
- Seizures, nausea and vomiting frequently occur.
- Often non-specific presentation. Cerebral venous sinus thrombosis should be considered in young patients with headache or stroke-like symptoms without any vascular risk factors.

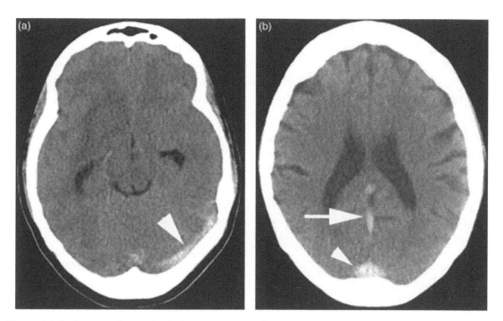

Figure 66 Axial images showing high-density acute thrombus within the (a) left transverse sinus (arrowhead); (b) straight sinus (arrow), and torcula (arrowhead).

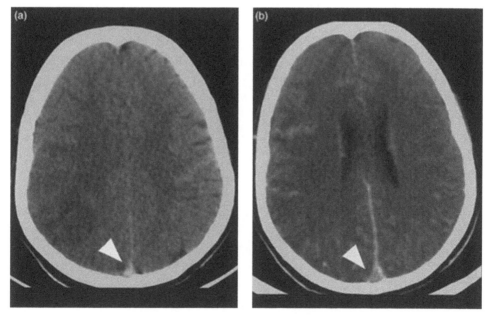

Figure 67 Axial images: (a) pre-contrast image showing hyperdense acute thrombus within the posterior sagittal sinus – the delta sign (arrowhead); (b) post-contrast image demonstrating contrast outlining the thrombus – the empty delta sign (arrowhead).

Radiological Features

CT

- CT scan without contrast should be performed initially to rule out haemorrhagic-related causes. This can then be followed by a contrast-enhanced scan.

Features

- CT may be normal.

Non-contrast CT

- Thrombus appears hyperdense for the first 7–14 days, after which it is isodense.
- Thrombus within a cerebral vein – linear hyperdense material within a vessel representing thrombosed blood (Fig. 66).
- Superior sagittal sinus thrombosis – classically hyperdense triangle within the sinus known as the '*delta sign*' (Fig. 67a).
- Low-attenuation areas of cerebral infarction not conforming to an arterial territory.

Contrast CT

- Thrombus will appear as a filling defect surrounded by enhancing dura.
- Superior sagittal sinus thrombosis – look for the '*empty delta*' sign (seen in 70%) (Fig. 67b).
  - This is a filling defect within the straight/superior sagittal sinus, and represents flow around a non-enhanced clot.
- Gyral enhancement peripheral to an infarction in 30–40%.
- Coexisting signs of infection or inflammation (e.g. sinusitis/mastoiditis) should raise suspicion.

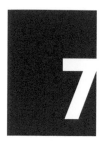

Hypoxic–Ischaemic Injury (HII)

Characteristics
- Results from all causes leading to diminished cerebral blood flow (ischaemia) and reduced blood oxygenation (hypoxaemia).
- Affects all age groups, from premature infants to adults. The pattern of damage is determined by the degree of brain maturity, metabolic activity in the area of affected brain, severity and duration of the hypoxic ischaemic insult.
- Asphyxia is the most common cause in infants, with cardiac arrest being the leading cause in adults.
- A devastating condition, which can result in severe long-term neurological disability and death.
- Imaging helps to secure an early diagnosis, enabling intervention in the acute stage. Information on severity and extent of injury in the subacute setting helps to predict long-term outcome.

Clinical Features
Term and Preterm Neonates
- Related to antepartum (maternal hypotension, multiple gestations and prenatal infection) or intrapartum risk factors (forceps delivery, breech extraction or placental abruption).
- Premature neonates are more vulnerable to perinatal insults leading to hypoperfusion.
- Imaging plays an important role in distinguishing between neurological immaturity and HII, as clinical signs can be confusing.

Children and Adults
- HII in adults often results from cardiac arrest or cerebrovascular disease.
- Drowning and asphyxiation are the more common causes in older children.

Post-anoxic Leukoencephalopathy
- A specific but uncommon cause of delayed white matter injury occurring weeks after the hypoxic–ischaemic event, most commonly associated with carbon monoxide poisoning.
- Can also manifest as progressive deterioration in neurology.

- Delirium, personality changes, intellectual impairment, movement disorders or seizures may be present.

Radiological Features

CT

- Early CT may appear 'normal' with subtle low-density change in the deep grey matter.
- Subsequent changes include cortical hypoattenuation, loss of normal grey/white matter differentiation and diffuse cerebral oedema, with cisternal and sulcal effacement.
- The *'reversal sign'* may be seen within the first 24 hours, with higher attenuation of the white matter compared with the cortical grey matter.
- The *'white cerebellum sign'*, caused by diffuse oedema, may be observed resulting in hypoatteunation of the cerebral hemispheres with sparing of the cerebellum and brainstem (Fig. 68).

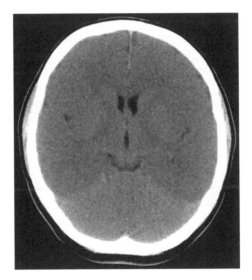

Figure 68 Axial CT brain image demonstrating complete loss of cerebral grey/white matter differentiation, with relative increase in attenuation of the cerebellum, due to diffuse oedema of the cerebral hemispheres – white cerebellum sign.

Skull Fractures

Characteristics

- Result from trauma to the head.
- Classified as linear, depressed or base of skull fractures.
- Linear fractures are often uncomplicated and do not require treatment.
- However, temporal bone fractures may result in an extradural haematoma.
- Depressed skull fractures may require surgery to elevate the bone fragments to prevent brain injury.
- Increased significance if the fracture is open, or communicates with an adjacent sinus, due to increased risk of infection.
- In basal skull fractures prophylactic antibiotics were once routinely prescribed to reduce the risk of meningitis, but their use is no longer routine.

Clinical Features

- Open fractures underlie scalp lacerations and are often diagnosed during evaluation of the wound for closure.
- Depressed skull fractures are often palpable or visible during examination, but may be masked by swelling around the area.
- Clinical signs of base of skull fracture:
    - CSF rhinorrhoea/otorrhoea.
    - Haemotympanum.
    - Bleeding from the external auditory meatus.
    - Racoon eyes.
    - Subconjunctival haemorrhage (with no posterior limit).
    - Battle's sign (bruising over the mastoid area).
    - Cranial nerve deficits.

Radiological Features

CT

- Look closely at the initial scout image as this may demonstrate a fracture.
- Soft tissue swelling, or an underlying brain abnormality, may be associated with a fracture.
- Fractures may be missed if appropriate 'window' parameters are not chosen. Always assess for fractures on bony windows.
- Fractures appear as sharply defined lines (Figs. 69–72)and should not be mistaken for a suture or vascular groove; a vascular groove often branches and both have typical sites.

- The presence of intracranial air may be secondary to an open fracture or connection with an air-containing sinus.
- Modern reconstruction techniques, e.g. multiplanar and surface rendering (Fig. 75), are useful to delineate fracture anatomy.

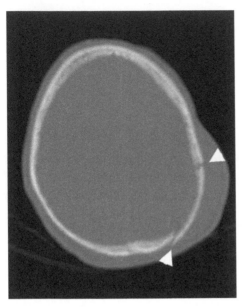

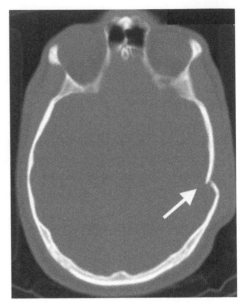

Figure 69 Left parietal bone fracture (arrowheads) with marked overlying soft tissue contusion.

Figure 70 Depressed skull fracture (arrow).

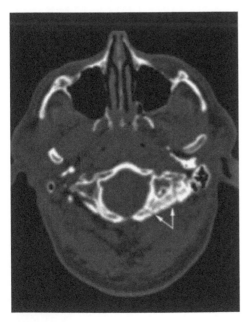

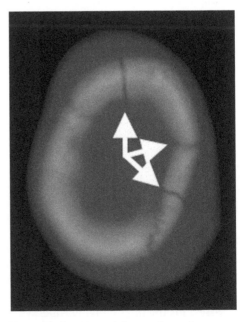

Figure 71 Base of skull fracture (arrows).

Figure 72 Complex vault fracture (arrows).

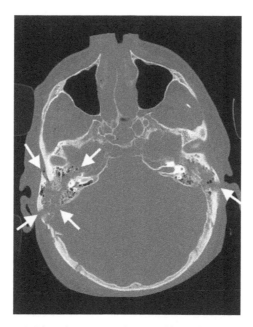

Figure 73 Bilateral comminuted temporal bone fractures (arrows).

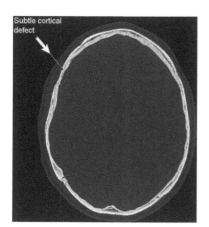

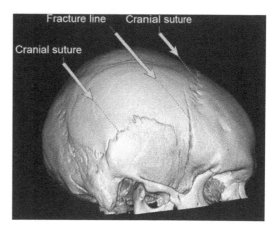

Figure 74 A subtle cortical defect is seen in the right frontal bone (arrow). This could be followed cranicaudally on adjacent axial images (not shown). Care should be taken not to misinterpret this as a suture. Surface-rendered images can be helpful in distinguishing between a fracture and a cranial suture.

Figure 75 Surface-rendered image of a skull fracture (same patient discussed in Fig. 74). The fracture line is much more readily identifiable from the adjacent cranial suture.

Raised Intracranial Pressure

Characteristics

- The skull defines a fixed volume.
- A relatively small increase in volume can lead to a disproportionate rise in intracranial pressure (ICP).
- As ICP increases, ultimately cerebral perfusion pressure (CPP) decreases.
- Once CPP is < 70 mmHg, significant brain injury can occur.
- CPP is autoregulated by pCO_2 receptors. Current guidance recommends maintaining pCO_2 towards the lower end of the normal range in a brain-injured patient.
- Raised ICP yields an increase in systemic arterial blood pressure and a bradycardia – this is called the *Cushing Response.*
- Causes of raised intracranial pressure include:
  - Haemorrhage (subdural, epidural, subarachnoid, intracerebral, intraventricular).
  - Brain abscess.
  - Meningoencephalitis.
  - Primary or metastatic tumours.
  - Hydrocephalus.
  - Cerebral oedema (vasogenic, cytotoxic or interstitial).

Clinical Features

- Patients often present with a vague history of listlessness, irritability, drowsiness, +/– nausea and vomiting.
- Early morning headaches or a headache that wakens from sleep should be considered as sinister.
- The presentation may be acute with sudden neurological deterioration.
- Third nerve palsy – dilated ipsilateral pupil and ophthalmoplegia develop as ICP rises.
- Papilloedema is an unreliable sign. Look for absence of venous pulsation.
- Classic progression of symptoms:
  - Bradycardia with associated rising blood pressure (Cushing Response).
  - Respiratory depression.
  - Pupillary constriction and then dilation.

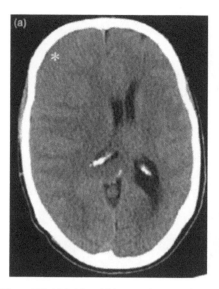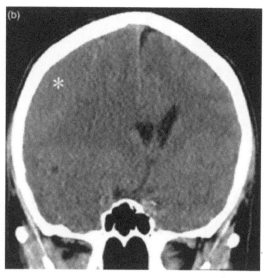

Figure 76 (a) Axial and (b) coronal images showing subfalcine hernation secondary to mass effect from subacute subdural haematoma (asterix).

Radiological Features

- CSF spaces are reduced in size with effacement of sulci and the basal cisterns.
- Herniation of brain parenchyma (representing shift of the normal brain, through or across regions, to another site due to mass effect) occurs late.

Brain Herniation

- *Subfalcine herniation* (Fig. 76) – displacement of the cingulate gyrus across the midline under the falx. The anterior cerebral artery is displaced resulting in secondary ischaemia and infarction.
- *Transtentorial herniation* (Fig. 77) – downward displacement of temporal lobes and brain stem leading to effacement of the basal cisterns, dilatation of the contralateral ventricular system due to obstruction to CSF flow and midline shift of the brain parenchyma.
- *Tonsillar herniation* (Fig. 78) – cerebellar tonsils are displaced inferiorly through the foramen magnum. Look for loss of the low-density CSF fluid around the brainstem at this level.

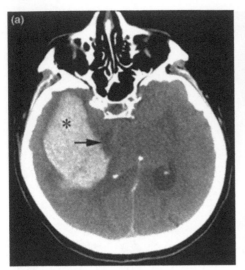
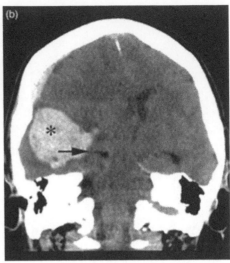

Figure 77 (a) Axial and (b) coronal images showing transtentorial herniation with effacement of the basal cisterns secondary to a right intraparenchymal haematoma (asterix). Black arrow indicates the medially displaced temporal horn of the right lateral ventricle. There is also evidence of subfalcine herniation and a right-sided subdural haematoma.

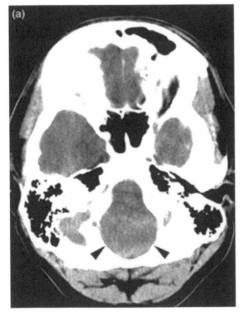
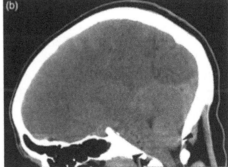

Figure 78 (a) Axial and (b) sagittal images showing tonsillar herniation with complete effacement of the CSF space at the level of the foramen magnum (arrowheads).

10 Hydrocephalus

Characteristics

Hydrocephalus is an accumulation of CSF in the brain, which results from an imbalance between CSF production and absorption.

- Communicating hydrocephalus.

  Reduced CSF absorption.

  - · Obstruction at the level of pacchionian granulations.
  - · SAH, meningitis, venous thrombosis.

  Increased CSF production.

  - · Choroid plexus tumours.

  Normal pressure hydrocephalus.

  - · Clinical triad: gait disturbance, dementia and urinary incontinence.
  - · No evidence of raised intracranial pressure.
  - · Non-communicating hydrocephalus.

- Obstruction of the ventricles, foraminae or aqueduct, causing dilatation proximal to the obstruction with normal calibre distal to the obstruction.

Causes

- *Foramen of Monro.*
  - · Colloid cyst of the third ventricle, oligodendroglioma, ependymoma, suprasellar tumours, giant cell astrocytoma (tuberous sclerosis).
- *Aqueduct of Sylvius.*
  - · Congenital aqueduct stenosis, intraventricular haemorrhage, ventriculitis.
- *Fourth ventricle/foraminae of Luschka and Magendie.*
  - · Congenital: Dandy–Walker malformation, intraventricular haemorrhage, posterior fossa tumours: ependymoma, medulloblastoma, haemangioblastoma.

Clinical Features

- Neonate/infant.
  - Enlarged cranium, bulging fontanelles, widely separated cranial sutures, vomiting, drowsiness, irritability, eyes turned downwards due to paralysis of upward gaze.
- Older children and adults.
  - Headaches, nausea, vomiting, papilloedema, diplopia, problems with balance and coordination, gait disturbance, urinary incontinence.

Radiological Features

CT

Communicating Hydrocephalus

- Symmetrical enlargement of the ventricles.
- Mass effect causing effacement of sulci.
- Periventricular interstitial oedema.

Non-communicating Hydrocephalus

- Disproportionate dilatation of the ventricles proximal to the obstruction.
- Abnormality causing the obstruction (Fig. 79).

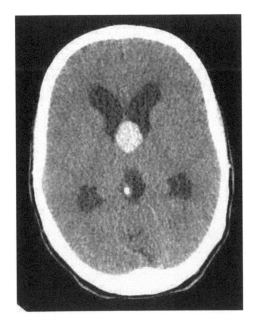

Figure 79 Axial image showing obstructive hydrocephalus, secondary to a hyperdense colloid cyst at the level of the foramen of Monro. There is resultant mass effect with dilatation of both frontal horns and trigones of the lateral ventricles, and generalised effacement of the cerebral sulci.

- Dilated temporal horns of the lateral ventricles (Fig. 82).
- Mass effect causing effacement of the sulci.
- Periventricular low-attenuation interstitial oedema from venous congestion (Fig. 80 and Fig. 81).

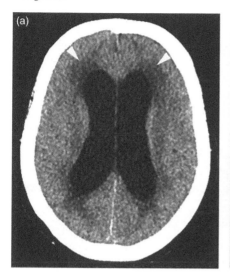 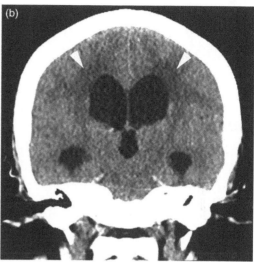

Figure 80 (a) Axial and (b) coronal images showing symmetrical dilatation of the lateral ventricles, and ballooning of the third ventricle. There is periventricular low-attenuation interstitial oedema (arrowheads). Note also generalised effacement of the extra-axial spaces.

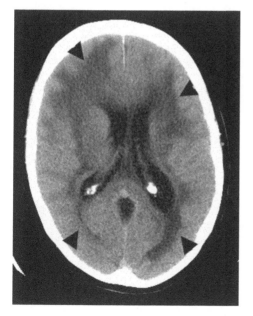 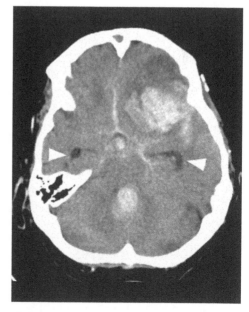

Figure 81 Acute hydrocephalus: periventricular low attenuation is seen (arrowheads) representing interstitial oedema from transependymal flow of CSF.

Figure 82 Acute parenchymal, subarachnoid and intraventricular haemorrhage, with resultant dilatation of the temporal horns (arrowheads) due to developing communicating hydrocephalus.

Meningitis

Characteristics

- Inflammation of the meninges, which can be further divided anatomically into:
  - *Pachymeningitis* – inflammation of the dura.
  - *Leptomeningitis* – inflammation of the arachnoid membrane and subarachnoid space.
  - *Meningoencephalitis* – inflammation extending to involve the parenchyma.
- Widespread use of the haemophilus influenzae B, pneumococcal and meningococcal C vaccines have reduced the incidence of meningitis in children.
- The median age of patients has risen to 25 years and it has become a disease of young adults.
- Concurrent illness such as pneumonia or other sites of sepsis (e.g. sinusitis, mastoiditis, otitis media) may extend directly to involve the meninges.

Clinical Features

- Presentation with fever, stiff neck, photophobia, headache and cerebral dysfunction, although common, is not specific for meningitis.
- Kernig's and Brudzinski's signs indicate the presence of meningeal irritation.
- Seizures, cranial nerve palsies and signs of raised ICP, such as papilloedema and Cushing reflex, may also be present.
- Detection at the extremes of age is difficult. Children may present with poor feeding, irritability, lethargy and vomiting. The elderly may only have a low-grade fever and delirium.
- CSF sampling for Gram stain, white cell count, glucose and protein will confirm the diagnosis. CT of the head is required prior to lumbar puncture in the presence of depressed consciousness or focal neurological deficit.

Radiological Features

CT

- CT scan without contrast should be performed in the first instance to rule out a haemorrhagic cause of the symptoms.

Features

Non-contrast CT

- Often normal in the early phase.
- Subtle meningeal thickening with increased density may be present.
- Features of secondary complications such as abscess, cerebral oedema, raised ICP, hydrocephalus and venous sinus thrombosis may be present.
- Reduction in size of the basal and suprasellar cisterns with sulcal effacement is suggestive of cerebral oedema and raised ICP.
- A primary infective source may be identified in the study, e.g. sinusitis and mastoiditis. Check on bone windows for bone destruction.

Contrast-enhanced CT

- Enhancement of the meningeal surfaces is non-specific, and is often an inconsistent finding in patients with meningitis. Best seen over the cerebral convexities and in the interhemispheric and Sylvian fissures (Fig. 83).
- Intense contrast enhancement of the thickened meninges, noted on the non-contrast CT, is suggestive of granulomatous meningitis, as seen in tuberculosis (TB) or sarcoidosis.

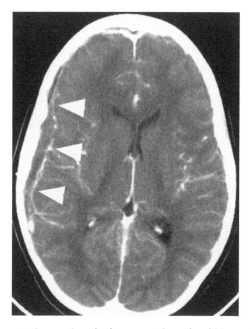

Figure 83 Axial image demonstrating meningeal enhancement (arrowheads) in a patient with pneumococcal meningitis, with a concurrent subdural empyema.

Cerebral Abscess

Characteristics
- Localised purulent bacterial infection developing in an area of cerebritis.

Causes
- Septic emboli transmitted haematogenously (e.g. secondary to endocarditis).
- Transdural spread from adjacent sinus infection.
- Penetrating trauma or surgery.

Predisposing Factors
- Diabetes mellitus, steroids/immunosuppressive therapy, immune deficiency.

Causative Organisms
- Anaerobic *Streptococcus* (most common), *Staphylococcus, Bacteroides*.
- Multiple organisms in 20%.
- *Mycobacterium/Salmonella* are more common in developing countries.
- Toxoplasmosis in immunocompromised patients.

Clinical Features
- Headache, vomiting, seizures, altered mental state and spiking pyrexia.
- Cranial nerve palsies or localised peripheral neurological deficits.
- Signs of raised ICP.
- Identifiable source of sepsis or pyrexia of unknown origin.
- Diagnosis and treatment is difficult in those who are immunosuppressed.
- Significant long-term morbidity.

Radiological Features

CT
- Initial CT scan should be performed without contrast to rule out a haemorrhagic cause of symptoms. Subsequent scan with contrast can then be performed.

Features

- Typically at the corticomedullary junction in the frontal and temporal lobes.

Non-contrast CT

- Low-attenuation lesion with associated mass effect.
- Gas within the lesion from gas-forming organisms.

Contrast-enhanced CT

- Thin-walled ring enhancement (2–7 mm) with a smooth convex surface (Fig. 84) (compared with a thick, irregular wall in a cerebral neoplasm).
- Central low-attenuation necrosis, which does not fill with contrast.
- Surrounding low-attenuation oedema causing mass effect.
- Lesions may be multiloculated and adjacent daughter abscesses may develop.
- Extension into the ventricles can result in ventriculitis. This is confirmed by increase in attenuation of CSF fluid within the ventricles with associated ependymal enhancement (Fig. 85).

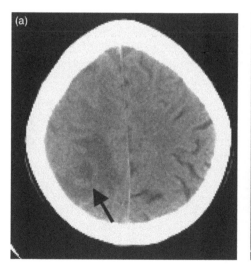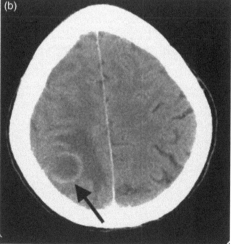

Figure 84 Axial CT images: (a) pre-contrast and (b) post-contrast, showing right superior parietal ring enhancing lesion (black arrows) with surrounding vasogenic oedema.

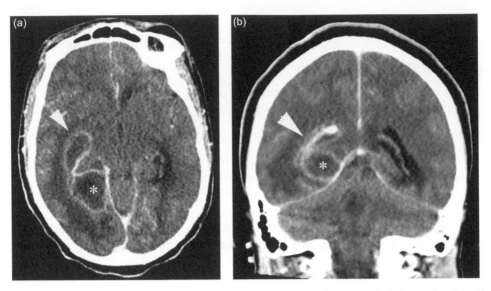

Figure 85 Post-contrast (a) axial and (b) coronal CT images showing a right intracerebral abscess (asterix) with rim enhancement; note the ependymal enhancement in the adjacent ventricle in keeping with ventriculitis (arrowhead).

Arteriovenous Malformation

13

Characteristics

- Congenital abnormality secondary to failure of embryonic vascular plexus differentiation.
- Cerebral vascular lesions allow low-pressure direct shunting of blood from the arterial to the venous system, without an intervening capillary bed, resulting in enlarged feeding vessels and draining veins.
- Accounts for 11% of cerebrovascular malformations and may be part of a congenital syndrome, e.g. Sturge–Weber, neurofibromatosis or von Hippel–Lindau syndrome.
- Venous malformations are less common, e.g. medullary venous and cavernous malformations. Arteriovenous fistulae are usually post-traumatic.

Clinical Features

- Often asymptomatic and clinically silent until the presenting event, although 10% are diagnosed incidentally.
- Minor cognitive impairment in up to two-thirds of patients, although largely subclinical and often do not come to medical attention.
- Headaches may be reported in up to half of all patients and may take the form of migraines.
- May present with seizures (non-focal in 40%), acute intracranial haemorrhage or progressive neurological deficit. Rarely, focal neurological deficit may indicate the site of an AVM.

Radiological Features

CT

- Non-contrast CT should be used initially, as high-density contrast may mask underlying haemorrhage.

Location

- Supratentorial (90%): parietal > frontal > temporal > occipital lobe.
- Infratentorial (10%).

Vascular Supply

- Pial branches of the internal carotid artery (ICA) in 75% of supratentorial lesions and in 50% of posterior fossa lesions.
- Dural branches of the external carotid artery (ECA) in 25% of infratentorial lesions.

Features

Unenhanced CT

- Cerebral or extra-axial haemorrhage. Secondary signs of AVM, including dilated dural sinuses and draining cerebral veins may be seen, although these are better demonstrated post contrast.
- 10% of AVM are not visualised on unenhanced CT.
- Lesions can appear as an isoattenuating to hyperattenuating mass:
  - *Mixed-density lesion* (60%), composed of large dense vessels, haemorrhage and calcification (Fig. 86).
  - *Isodense lesion* (15%), which may only be recognisable by associated mass effect.
  - *Low-density lesion* (15%), due to encephalomalacia, atrophy or gliosis secondary to associated local cerebral ischaemia.

Contrast-enhanced CT

- AVMs may enhance, with dense serpiginous enhancement representing tortuous dilated vessels in 80% of cases (Fig. 87).
- Adjacent low attenuation may be present due to oedema, mass effect or ischaemic changes.

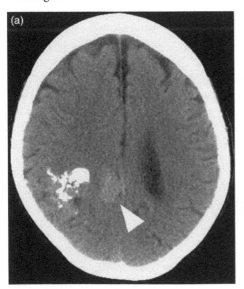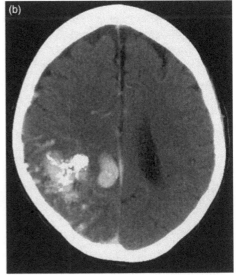

Figure 86 Axial CT images: (a) pre-contrast and (b) post-contrast, showing a mixed-density lesion composed of coarse calcification and faintly hyperdense vessels (arrowhead). There is marked enhancement within the tortuous vessels post-contrast.

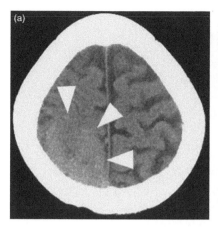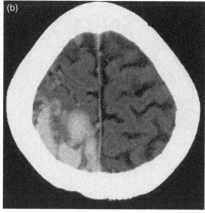

Figure 87 Axial CT images: (a) pre-contrast and (b) post-contrast showing large, faintly hyperdense cortical vessels seen at the right vertex (arrowheads) with marked enhancement post-contrast.

CT Angiography

Features

- Demonstrates the presence of a nidus and venous shunting to confirm diagnosis.
- Despite advances in spatial and temporal resolution, delineation of feeding arteries and draining veins is technically difficult. Cerebral angiography is therefore required for haemodynamic assessment and treatment planning.

Solitary Lesions

14

Characteristics

- Solitary space-occupying lesions are frequently tumours.
- One-third are metastases from breast, lung or melanoma primaries.
- Most commonly found in the cerebral hemisphere at the grey–white matter junction.
- Primary tumours (e.g. astrocytoma, glioblastoma multiforme, oligodendrogliomas, ependymomas) have < 50% 5-year survival. Two-thirds are supratentorial in adults, while two-thirds are infratentorial in children.
- Other solitary lesions included in the differential diagnosis are cerebral abscesses, aneurysms, tuberculomas, granulomas and cysts.

Clinical Features

- Seizures are a common first presentation in adults.
- Focal neurology may evolve with increasing size of the lesion or associated mass effect.
- Tumours usually run an indolent course and rarely cause a sudden increase in intracranial pressure.
- Solitary mass lesions can cause local effects, e.g. proptosis or epistaxis.
- Clinical presentation may help localise the site of the lesion:
  - *Frontal lobe* – hemiparesis, seizures, personality change, grasp reflex (unilateral is significant), expressive dysphasia (Broca's area) and anosmia.
  - *Temporal lobe* – complex partial seizures, hallucinations, feelings of déjà vu, taste, smell, dysphasia (Wernicke's area), visual field defects, fugue, functional psychosis.
  - *Parietal lobe* – hemisensory loss, decreased stereognosis, sensory inattention, dysphasia and Gerstmann's syndrome (finger agnosia, left/right disorientation, dysgraphia, acalculia).
  - *Occipital lobe* – contralateral visual field defects.
  - *Cerebellum* – past-pointing, intention tremor, nystagmus, dysdiadochokinesis and truncal ataxia (worse if eyes open).
  - *Cerebellopontine angle* – nystagmus, reduced corneal reflex, fifth and seventh cranial nerve palsies, ipsilateral cerebellar signs and ipsilateral deafness.
  - *Mid-brain* – unequal pupils, confabulation, somnolence and an inability to direct the eyes up or down.

Radiological Features

CT

Features

- The age of the patient and lesion location will aid the differential diagnosis, although often not vital in the emergency setting.
- Cerebral masses encompass a spectrum of appearances (Table 1):
  - *Density*: lesions may be hypo-, iso- or hyperdense.
  - *Calcification*: if present, may indicate a less aggressive pathology.
  - *Contrast enhancement*: often helpful in lesion characterisation. In cases of rim enhancement, abscess should be excluded (Fig. 88).
- Important to identify complications such as haemorrhage, cerebral oedema, hydrocephalus and cerebellar tonsillar herniation.

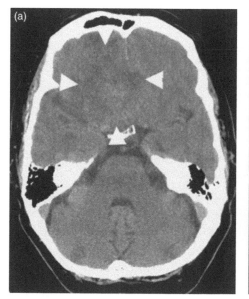 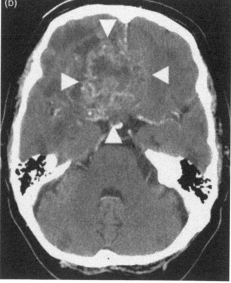

Figure 88 Frontal glioma: (a) pre-contrast and (b) post-contrast axial images showing ill-defined areas of low attenuation within the right frontal lobe (arrowheads). There is significant enhancement post contrast, with central low attenuation in keeping with necrosis. There is associated peripheral low-density oedema.

Table 1 CT imaging features of some commonly seen lesions.

Lesion	Location	Density	Calcification	Contrast enhancement
Haematoma < 1 week	Variable	↑	–	–
Haematoma 1–2 weeks	Variable	↔	–	–
Haematoma > 2 weeks	Variable	↓	Occasional	–
Colloid cysts	Foramen of Monro	↑ (80%)/ ↔ (20%)	–	Peripheral
Arachnoid cyst	Anterior temporal lobe (50%)	↓	–	–
Giant aneurysm	Cavernous/ supraclinoid ICA, basilar	↑	Curvilinear	Target sign
Pyogenic abscess	Variable	↓	–	Ring enhancement
Meningioma (Fig. 89)	Supratentorial (90%), extra-axial	↑ (70%)	Circular or radial	Intense uniform
Ependymoma (NF)	Floor of 4th ventricle	↔/ mildly ↑	Occasionally punctate	Solid component only
Primary lymphoma (HIV)	Periventricular, crosses the midline	↑	–	Homogeneous
Metastases	Corticomedullary junction, multiple	↓ (unless haemorrhagic)		Solid/ring-like
Glioblastoma multiforme (Fig. 90)	Frontal/temporal lobe, callosal	↓/↔/↑ (haemorrhage)	Rarely	Homo/ heterogeneous, ring pattern
Medulloblastoma	Cerebellum; vermis and roof of 4th ventricle	↑ (70%)	Rarely (13%)	Intense homogeneous
Vestibular schwannoma (NF2)	Cerebellopontine angle	↔/↓	–	Uniform dense/ ring-like
Haemangioblastoma (VHL)	Paravermian cerebellar hemisphere (85%)	↓ (cystic)	–	Peripheral mural/ solid enhancing
Epidermoid	Cerebellopontine angle (40%)	↓	25%	25% Peripheral
Dermoid	Posterior fossa (vermis)/4th ventricle	↓ (fat content)	Mural/central	–
Craniopharyngioma	Multilobular suprasellar (50%)	↔ (54–75%)	Marginal	Peripheral if cystic/ enhances if solid

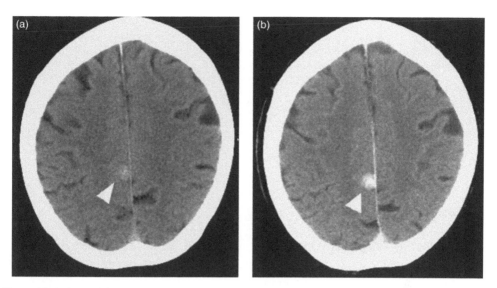

Figure 89 Right parafalcine meningioma: (a) pre-contrast and (b) post-contrast axial images showing a faintly hyperdense extra-axial lesion prior to contrast, which enhances avidly post-contrast (arrowhead).

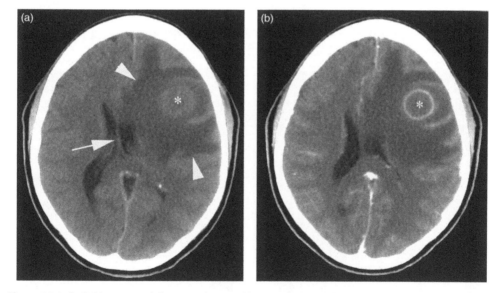

Figure 90 Left glioblastoma multiforme: axial images (a) pre-contrast and (b) post-contrast showing a left frontal lesion (asterix) with extensive surrounding oedema (arrowheads). There is significant mass effect with midline shift to the right (arrow) and avid rim enhancement post-contrast.

Multiple Lesions

15

Characteristics

- The differential diagnosis of multiple lesions include:
  - *Neoplastic:* Metastases (Figs. 91 and 92a–c) are the most common intracerebral neoplastic lesion (lung, breast, melanoma, renal, colon primaries). Found in up to 24% of all patients who die from cancer. Represents 20–30% of all brain tumours in adults.
  - *Infective:* cerebral abscesses (Fig. 93a,b), granulomata (Fig. 92d).
  - *Vascular:* multiple lesions of varying age are seen in multi-infarct dementia.
  - *Inflammatory:* demyelinating plaques can be seen as multiple low-density lesions on CT, predominantly in the periventricular deep white matter.
  - *Traumatic:* contusions are frequently multiple after head trauma.

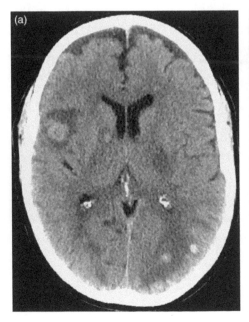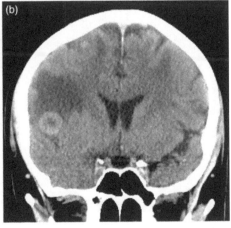

Figure 91 (a) Axial and (b) coronal unenhanced CT images demonstrating multiple hyperdense lesions with marked surrounding vasogenic oedema. Appearances are in keeping with metastases from melanoma.

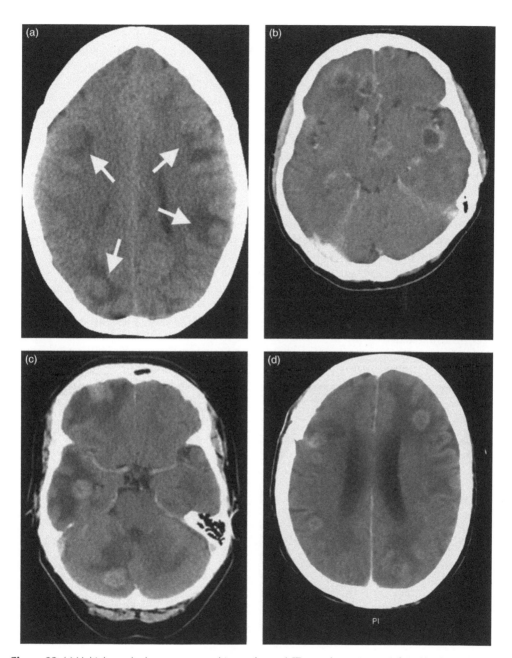

Figure 92 (a) Multiple cerebral metastases: on this unenhanced CT scan, the position is inferred by the associated oedema (arrows). (b) Multiple necrotic metastases with thick irregular rim enhancement. (c) Multiple solid enhancing metastases with surrounding vasogenic oedema. (d) Multiple tuberculomas showing thick irregular rim enhancement.

Clinical and Radiological Features

- Dependent on the underlying pathology. Please refer to Chapter 14 (Solitary lesions).

Radiological Features

CT

- Damage to the blood–brain barrier results in varying degrees of lesion enhancement. The pattern of enhancement may narrow the differential diagnosis.
- Melanoma metastases classically appear hyperdense prior to contrast enhancement (Fig. 91).
- Calcification in malignant tumours is uncommon. If present, this suggests metasteses from mucinous tumours of the gastrointestinal (GI) tract or breast, or cartilage/bone-forming sarcomas. Haemorrhage into metastases occurs infrequently, and when present suggests hypervascular tumours such as melanoma or renal cell carcinoma.
- Calcification following granulomatous infection is not uncommon.
- Cerebral contusions may be rather inconspicuous on initial CT, usually becoming more apparent on interval CT at about 2 weeks.
- MRI is much more sensitive in detecting contusions and should be considered if not contraindicated.

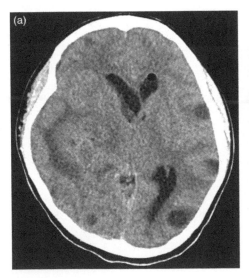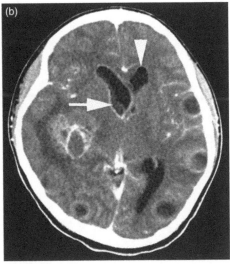

Figure 93 Axial CT images: (a) pre- and (b) post-contrast, demonstrating multiple low-attenuation ring-enhancing lesions. Note the high-attenuation material within the right frontal horn (arrow) and a gas locule within the left frontal horn (arrowhead); ependymal enhancement is seen in the right lateral ventricle. The overall appearance is in keeping with multiple cerebral abscesses.

16 Neck Vessel Dissection

Characteristics

- Dissection is defined as elevation or separation of arterial wall layers, most commonly the intima, from the underlying media.
- Begins as a tear in the arterial wall allowing flowing blood, under arterial pressure, to enter and separate the layers, thus creating a false lumen. This results in potential ischaemia from arterial stenosis or occlusion.
- The resulting intimal hematoma, +/− aneurysm formation, is a source of micro-emboli and can lead to further cerebral ischaemia.
- Accounts for up to 25% of strokes in patients < 50 years of age.
- Arterial dissection most commonly involves the carotid artery, and may affect both the extracranial and intracranial portions; the latter is more commonly involved, and often occurs just cranial to the bifurcation. Vertebral artery dissection occurs less frequently, and most commonly involves the extra-osseous segment at the C1–C2 level.
- Preceding trauma is common, and may be trivial, although spontaneous dissection can also occur. Other risk factors include hypertension and genetically related connective tissue disorders (Marfan syndrome, Ehlers–Danlos syndrome type IV and fibromuscular dysplasia). These may play a greater role in cases of minor trauma.

Clinical Features

- Presentation may be non-specific and a high index of suspicion is critical.
- Severe constant head, neck and facial pain are common (75%).
- Partial Horner syndrome (miosis, enopthalmus and ptosis) is reported in carotid dissection.
- The majority (93%) of patients will have focal neurological deficit related to an ischaemic stroke at the time of diagnosis; this can be delayed for several weeks in extracranial dissection.
- Other signs of maxillofacial trauma, cervical spine injury, hanging or strangulation should alert clinicians to this associated injury.

Radiological Features

CT Angiography

- CT angiography is sensitive and accurate for rapid and non-invasive diagnosis.
    - 100 ml of iodinated contrast injected via a pump, at 3–5 ml/sec, with coverage from the aortic arch to the circle of Willis; injection should be bolus-timed with a region of interest over the aortic arch.
- Study should be reviewed in axial slices, with multiplanar reformats and maximum intensity projections.

Features

- A thin, low-density intraluminal intimal flap may be seen, separating the high-density contrast within the lumen (Fig. 94).
- Centric or eccentric narrowing of the lumen may be observed. Associated crescentic thickening of the arterial wall is consistent with intramural haematoma.
- Absence of high-density contrast within the lumen suggests thrombosis and complete occlusion.
- Narrowing or dilatation of the calibre of the arterial lumen may also be observed.
- A careful search for associated injuries should be performed.

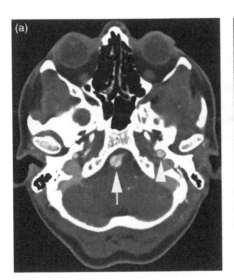 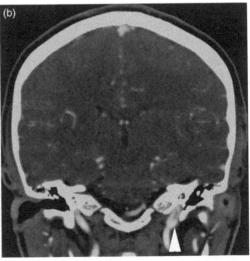

Figure 94 (a) Axial image of a CT angiogram, showing a dissection flap within the left internal carotid (arrowhead) and basilar (arrow) arteries. (b) Coronal image of a CT angiogram showing a left internal carotid artery dissection flap (arrowhead).

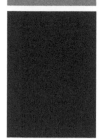

Cervical Spine

Characteristics

- The majority of cervical spine injuries are secondary to road traffic collisions.
- Falls from a height and sporting accidents make up the next largest categories.
- 50% of cervical spine injuries occur at C6 or C7.
- 33% of cervical spine injuries occur at C2.
- Cross-sectional imaging is performed when plain films are inadequate, if the cervical spine cannot be cleared clinically, or when there has been a significant mechanism of injury. Advancement and ease of access to CT has resulted in cross-sectional imaging being performed more frequently for cervical spine injuries.
- Plain film may identify potential ligamentous injury where abnormal flexion or extension occur on the lateral view – this should be correlated with clinical findings, and an MRI should be requested if clinically suspicious of ligamentous injury (Fig. 95 and 96).
- The aim of imaging is to identify an underlying injury, and to determine whether an injury is stable or unstable. Stability determines the management of the injury.

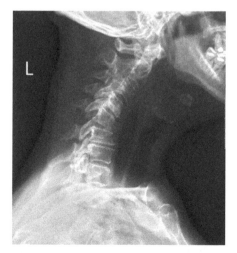

Figure 95 Lateral cervical spine radiograph demonstrating an acute kyphosis and retrolisthesis at C5/C6. There is significant widening of both the interspinous and facetal joint distances at this level. The appearances are in keeping with a highly unstable neck injury.

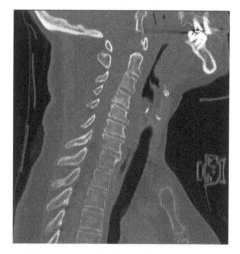

Figure 96 CT cervical spine (sagittal reformat) of same patient, performed to further evaluate the plain radiographic findings. Almost complete normalization of spinal alignment and only mild widening of the C5/C6 interspinous distance. This illustrates the potential limitations of CT in patients with a ligamentous injury.

- Local guidance will determine scan protocols. The scan should typically extend from the base of the skull to T6, and images should be reviewed axially in conjunction with sagittal and coronal reformats.
- The spinal column maintains its stability through a complex network of ligaments. In order to assess stability, the spine is divided into three distinct columns: anterior, middle and posterior.
  - The *anterior column* contains the anterior longitudinal ligament and the anterior two-thirds of the vertebral bodies, annulus fibrosus and intervertebral discs.
  - The *middle column* contains the posterior longitudinal ligament and the posterior third of the vertebral bodies, annulus and intervertebral discs.
  - The *posterior column* contains the bony elements formed by the pedicles, transverse processes, articulating facets, laminae and spinous processes.
- When one column is disrupted, the remaining two columns can provide sufficient stability to prevent spinal cord injury.
- When two or more columns are disrupted, the spinal column is regarded as unstable, as the spine can move as separate units, increasing the occurrence of spinal cord injury.

'ABCs' Approach to Interpreting Multiplanar Reformats of the CT Cervical Spine

A. Alignment

- Normal articulation of the craniocervical junction should be assessed on sagittal and axial planes; subluxation usually results from ligamentous injury.
- Normal smooth curves of the anterior vertebral, posterior vertebral and spino-laminar lines should be identified on the sagittal reconstruction, similar to interpretation of a lateral cervical spine radiograph (Fig. 97).
- In a child, pseudo-subluxation of C2 on C3 may be identified which can cause confusion. In these cases, examine the spinolaminar line from C1 to C3 on sagittal reconstructions. If the bases of the spinous processes lie greater than 2 mm from this line, an injury should be suspected. Correlate with soft-tissue findings (see below).
- The distance between the anterior arch of C1 and odontoid peg should be less than 3 mm in an adult and 5 mm in a child, measured on the mid-sagittal image, similar to the criteria used on a lateral radiograph.
- Facet joint alignment should be assessed on axial and sagittal images. The '*hamburger sign*' confirms normal alignment of the facet joint on axial images, with the two halves of the burger bun contributed to by the superior and inferior articular facets. In facet dislocation, the '*reverse hamburger sign*' is described where the orientation of the burger bun halves is reversed; the dislocation is apparent in the sagittal plane.
- The tips of the spinous processes should align in the midline in the coronal plane, similar to the appearances on an AP radiograph. Bifid spinous processes can make interpretation difficult.

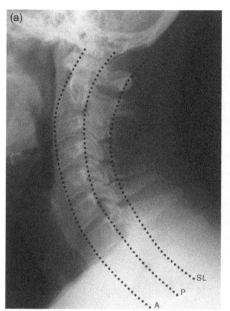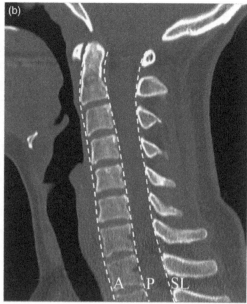

Figure 97 (a) Normal lateral radiography and (b) normal mid-sagittal CT cervical spine with three lines: anterior vertebral (A), posterior vertebral (P) and spinolaminar (SL) lines showing normal alignment.

B. Bone

- Vertebral bodies should be of uniform height, best assessed in sagittal and coronal planes. Increase in density or loss of vertebral height is in keeping with a compression fracture. Retro-pulsion of a fracture fragment into the spinal canal may result in spinal cord compression.
- Assess for the normal bony cortical outline. A breach in the cortex suggests a fracture; however, vascular channels also appear as lucent lines reaching the cortex and can be misinterpreted as a fracture. Correlation of these lines in all three planes helps to confirm the true presence of a fracture.

C. Cartilage

- The intervertebral spaces should be of uniform height in both sagittal and coronal planes.
- Widening of the intervertebral spaces, or interspinous distances, may indicate an unstable dislocation.
- An increase in the interspinous distance of greater than 50% suggests ligamentous disruption. Muscular spasm can make interpretation difficult.

S. Soft Tissues

- Retropharyngeal soft-tissue swelling may be the only sign of a significant injury; swelling takes time to form and may not be apparent if imaging is performed too early post-injury.
- Normal retropharyngeal measurements are less than 7 mm, anterior to C2–C4 (half a vertebral body width at this level) and less than 22 mm below C5 (one vertebral body width).
- Judicious assessment of structures surrounding the cervical spine is important to identify associated injuries. Examples include: mandibular fractures, temporomandibular joint subluxation/dislocation, injury to the aerodigestive tract, pneumomediastinum, ribs/sternum/scapula fractures and pneumothorax. This list is not exhaustive and careful interpretation is essential to ensure important injuries are not missed.
- Where spinal cord or ligamentous injury is suspected despite a normal CT, MRI or dynamic imaging should be performed to assess further.
- Cervical spine injuries can be classified according to the mechanism of injury (Fig. 98). These include flexion, flexion–rotation, extension, vertical compression and upper cervical spine injuries.

Types of Spine Fractures

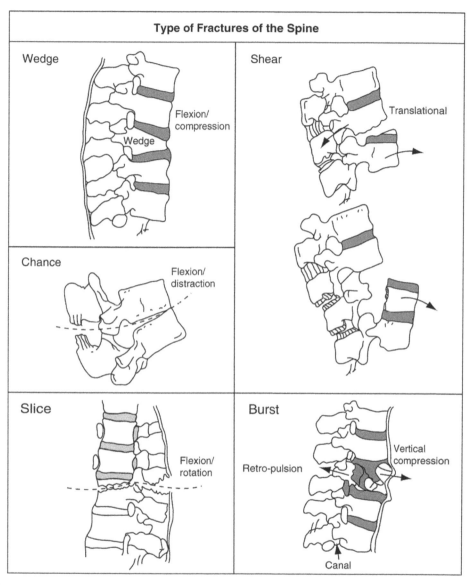

Figure 98 Diagram showing types of spine fracture. Types of fracture of the spine. From: *Sports Medicines: Problems and Practical Management* (Eds E. Sherry & D. Bokor); Greenwich Medical Media, 1997: p. 120.

The following tables classify the types of cervical spine injuries, their radiological features and stability.

Table 2 Flexion injuries.

Fracture type	Description and radiological features	Stability
Simple wedge compression fracture	Compression fracture of the antero-superior aspect of the vertebral body Prevertebral soft tissue swelling Reduced vertebral height anteriorly with increased concavity and sclerosis (secondary to impaction)	Stable unless associated with posterior ligamentous disruption (Fig. 99)
Flexion teardrop fracture (Fig. 100)	Flexion injury with vertical axial compression Fracture through the antero-inferior aspect of the vertebral body, often with anterior displacement of the fragment ('teardrop') Associated with significant ligamentous disruption All three columns are disrupted Associated with spinal cord injury (Differs from an extension teardrop fracture in that the anterior height of the vertebral body is usually reduced)	**Unstable**
Clay shoveller's fracture (Fig. 101)	Forced abrupt hyperflexion injury with neck and upper thoracic muscular contraction. Also caused by direct blow to the spinous processes Commonly occurs in the lower cervical/upper thoracic spine Oblique fracture of the base of a spinous process – avulsed by the supraspinous ligament Vertical split appearance of the spinous process on coronal view	Stable
Anterior subluxation	Posterior ligamentous complex ruptures and the anterior longitudinal ligament remains intact No associated bony injury Sagittal view – widening of interspinous distance. Anterior and posterior lines are disrupted in flexion views	Stable
Bilateral facet dislocation	Severe flexion injury from a large force The vertebral body above displaces anteriorly by at least 50% of the AP diameter of the vertebral body The inferior articulating facets of the upper vertebral body, moves superior and anterior to the superior articulating facets of the vertebral body below The facets often appear 'locked'. Associated with disc herniation	**Highly unstable**
Odontoid fracture (Fig. 102)	Type 1 occurs at the tip at the site of insertion of the alar ligament Type 2 involves the junction with the body of C2. Most common type of odontoid fracture. Associated with non-union due to limited blood supply & small area of cancellous bone. (Fig. 103) Type 3 extends into the body of C2. (Fig. 104)	Type 1 – stable Type 2 – **unstable** Type 3 – **unstable** if fragment separation
Uncinate process fracture	Lateral flexion injury	Stable

Types of Cervical Spine Fractures

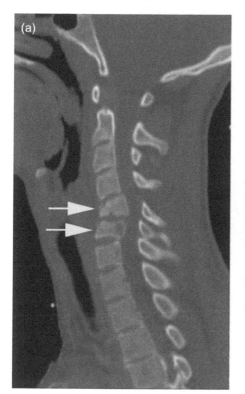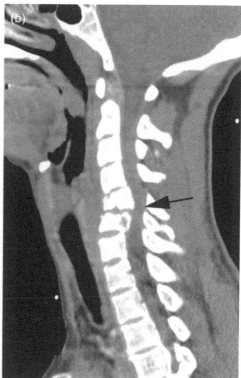

Figure 99 Sagittal CT images in (a) bone and (b) soft-tissue windows demonstrating loss of height of the C5 and C6 vertebral bodies, with retro-pulsion into the spinal canal (white arrows). Note the compression of the spinal cord demonstrated on soft-tissue windows (black arrow). The anterior and middle columns are disrupted; therefore, this represents an unstable injury.

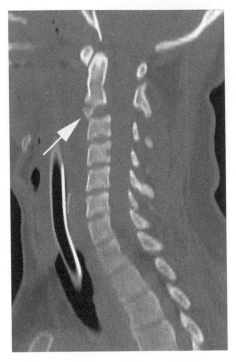

Figure 100 Sagittal CT image demonstrating fracture of the antero-inferior corner of the C2 vertebral body in keeping with flexion teardrop fracture.

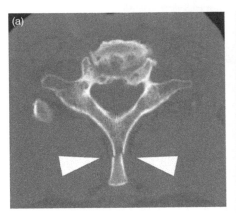
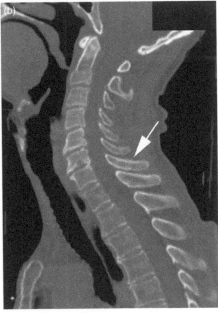

Figure 101 (a) Axial and (b) sagittal CT images demonstrating a fracture of the spinous process consistent with a clay shoveller's fracture.

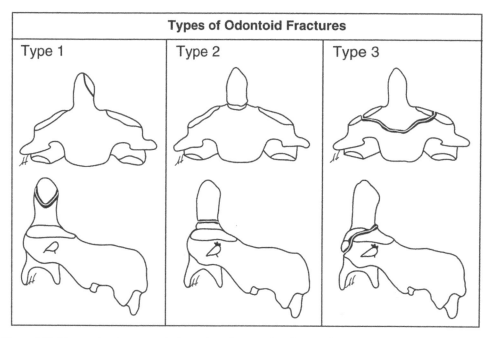

Figure 102 Diagram showing types of odontoid peg fractures. Classification of odontoid peg fractures. From: *Sports Medicines: Problems and Practical Management* (Eds E. Sherry & D. Bokor); Greenwich Medical Media, 1997: p. 117.

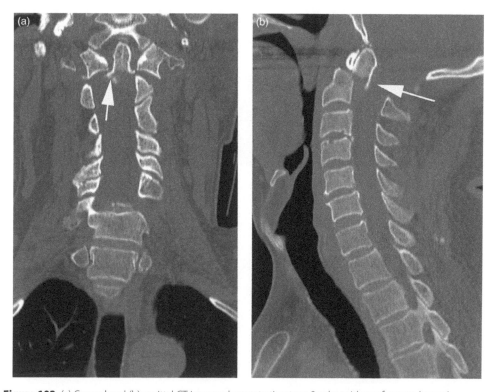

Figure 103 (a) Coronal and (b) sagittal CT images demonstrating type 2 odontoid peg fracture (arrows).

Table 3 Rotational injuries.

Fracture type	Description and radiological features	Stability
Unilateral facet dislocation. (Fig. 105)	Flexion/rotation injury One inferior articular facet of an upper vertebral body passes superior and anterior to the superior articular facet of the vertebral body below, and comes to rest in the intervertebral foramen The vertebral body above displaces anteriorly by less than 50% of the AP diameter of the vertebral body (compare with bilateral facet dislocation) Coronal view – disruption of the line joining the spinous processes at the level of the dislocation Oblique view – disruption of the typical shingles appearance at the level of the dislocation	Considered a stable injury unless it occurs at the C1/C2 level

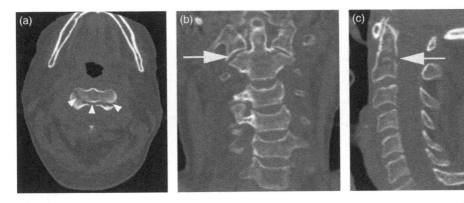

Figure 104 (a) Axial (arrowheads), (b) coronal and (c) sagittal CT images (arrows) demonstrating a type 3 odontoid peg fracture.

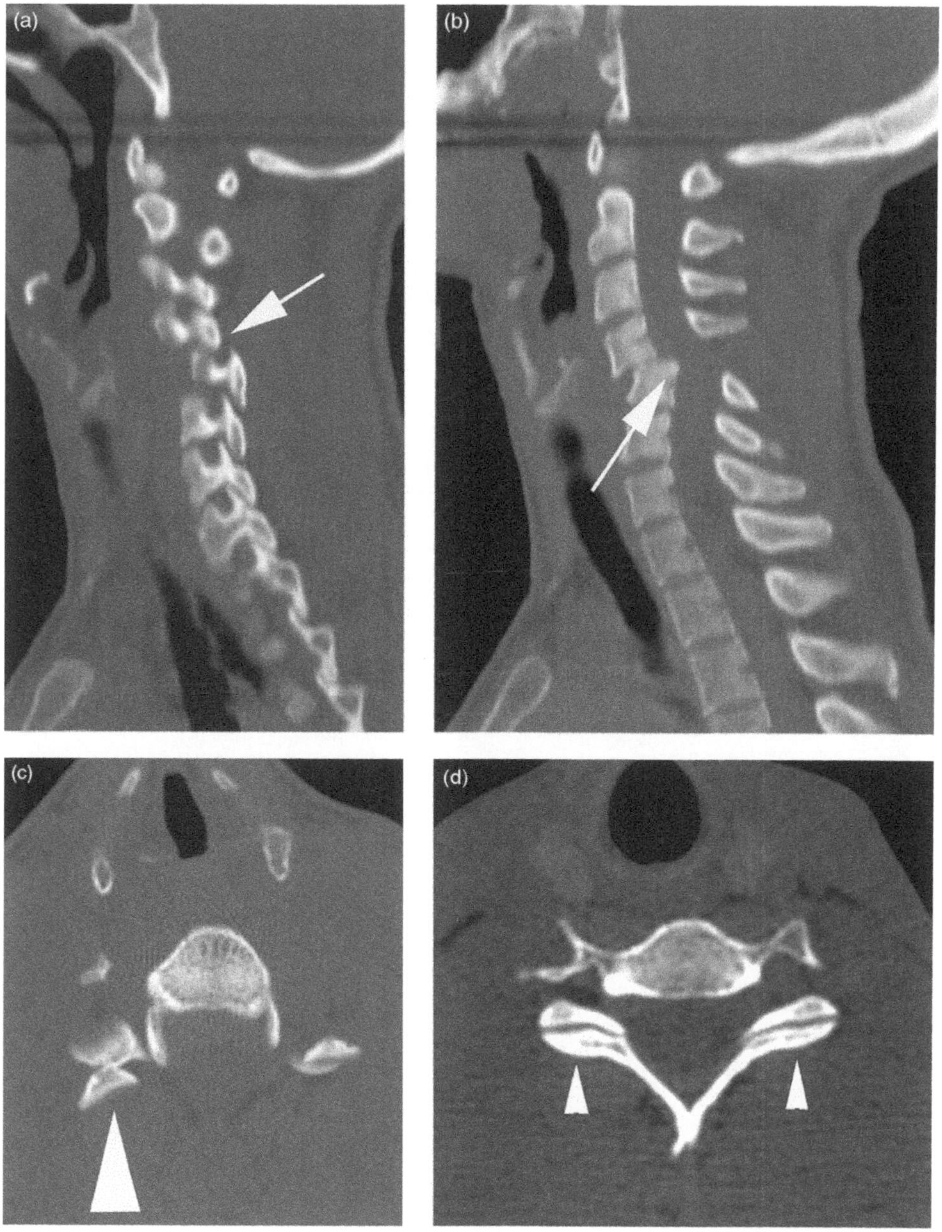

Figure 105 (a) Sagittal CT image demonstrating the inferior articular process of C4 passing anterosuperior to the superior articular facet of C5 (arrow). (b) Sagittal CT image showing loss of anterior and posterior vertebral alignment and posterior displacement of C5 into the spinal canal (arrow). (c) Axial CT image demonstrating the reverse hamburger sign, in facet dislocation (arrowhead); compare with (d) normal axial facet alignment (arrowheads).

Table 4 Extension injuries.

Fracture type	Description and radiological features	Stability
Fracture of posterior arch of the atlas	Hyperextension results in a compressive force, which compresses the posterior neural arch of the atlas between the occiput and the dens Sagittal view – fracture line through the posterior neural arch Coronal view – fails to show displacement of the lateral masses of C1 with respect to the articular pillars of C2 (thus distinguishing this fracture from a Jefferson fracture)	Stable
Extension teardrop fracture	Common in diving injuries and usually occurs at C5–C7 True avulsion injury with the anterior longitudinal ligament avulsing the antero-inferior corner of the vertebral body Vertebral body height is preserved May be associated with central cord syndrome with buckling of the ligamentum flavum	**Highly unstable**
Hangman's fracture (Fig. 106)	Traumatic bilateral fractures through the pedicles of C2 resulting in spondylolisthesis Common in road-traffic accidents. Fatal hangings result from a hyoid fracture and asphyxiation There is disruption of the spinolaminar line	**Unstable**

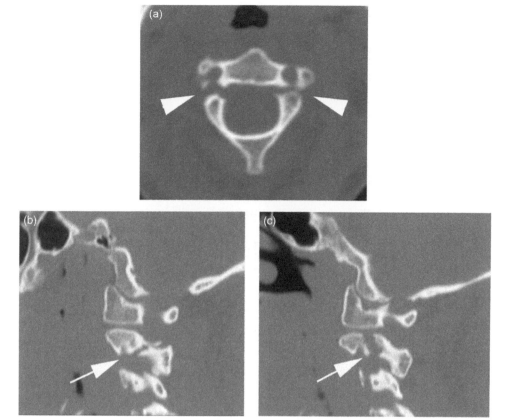

Figure 106 (a) Axial (arrowheads) and (b), (c) sagittal CT images (arrows) demonstrating fractures through the pedicles of C2 bilaterally in keeping with hangman's fracture.

Table 5 Vertebral compression injuries.

Fracture type	Description and radiological features	Stability
Jefferson fracture (Fig. 107)	Burst fracture of the ring of C1 A compressive force is transmitted evenly through the occipital condyles to the superior articular surfaces of the lateral masses of C1. The masses are forced laterally causing fractures of the anterior and posterior arches. There is usually disruption of the transverse ligament Sagittal view – significant soft tissue swelling Coronal odontoid view – unilateral or bilateral displacement of the lateral masses of C1 with respect to the articular pillars of C2	**Unstable**
Burst fracture	A downward compressive force is transmitted to lower vertebral bodies The intervertebral disc is driven into the vertebral body below causing it to shatter outwards Both anterior and middle columns are disrupted Comminuted vertebral body fracture with anterior and posterior displacement of fragments Fracture fragments may impinge on the cord causing anterior cord syndrome	**Unstable**

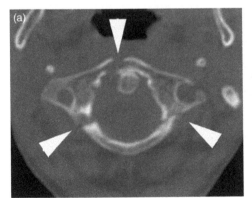 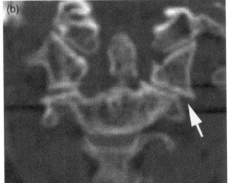

Figure 107 (a) Axial CT image demonstrating burst fractures affecting the anterior and posterior arches of C1 in keeping with a Jefferson burst fracture (arrowheads). (b) Coronal CT image demonstrating lateral displacement of the C1 lateral mass (arrow), similar to the appearances of a Jefferson burst fracture on the 'peg' view of C spine radiograph series. There is also a concurrent fracture of the odontoid peg.

Table 6 Upper cervical spine injuries.

Fracture	Description and radiological features	Stablility
Atlanto-occipital dislocation	Severe flexion or extension at the upper cervical level Involves complete disruption of all ligamentous relationships between the occiput and the atlas Death is often immediate due to stretching of the brainstem causing respiratory arrest There is disassociation between the base of the occiput and the arch of C1	**Highly unstable**
Atlanto-axial subluxation	Flexion injury without a lateral or rotatory component at the upper cervical level There is disruption of the transverse ligament There are shearing forces, as the skull grinds the atlanto-axial complex in flexion. Neurologic injury may occur from cord compression between the odontoid and posterior arch of C1 Sagittal view – predentate space > 3 mm in adults (> 5 mm in children)	**Highly unstable**

Self-assessment Section

Below are 12 random cases that vary in complexity from easy to difficult. This test is somewhat artificial as no clinical information is given and hence assessment is 'blind'. Formulate a provisional report and compare to the annotated answers at the end.

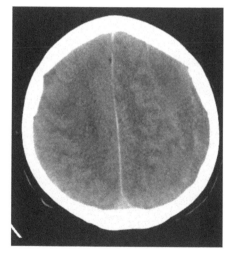

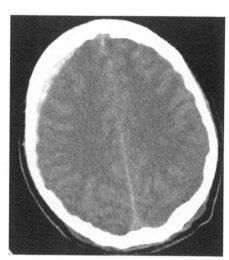

Case 1.   Case 2.

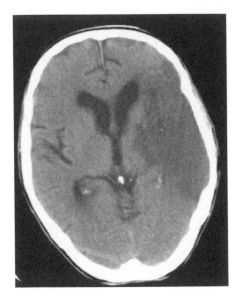

Case 3.

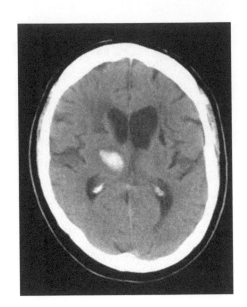

Case 4.

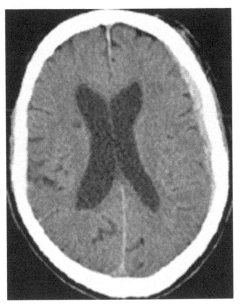

Case 5.

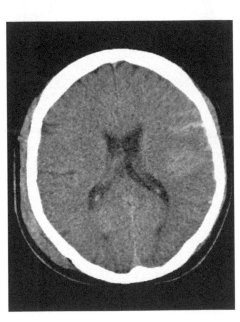

Case 6.

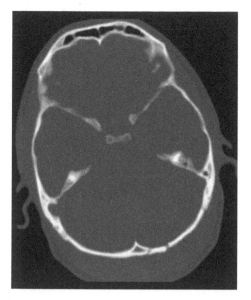

Case 7.

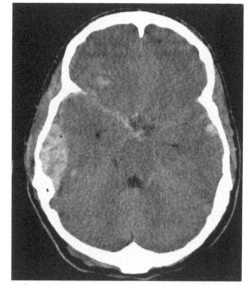

Case 8.

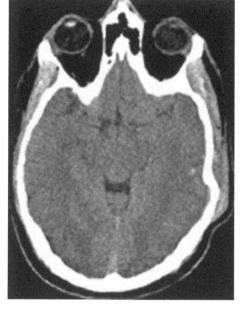

Case 9.

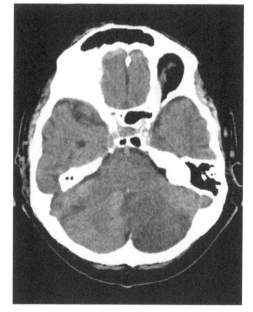

Case 10.

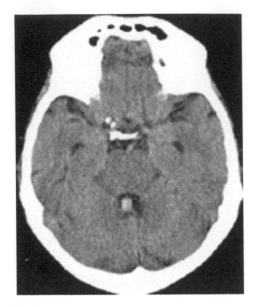

Case 11.

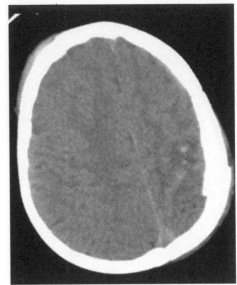

Case 12.

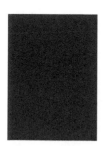

Self-assessment – Answers

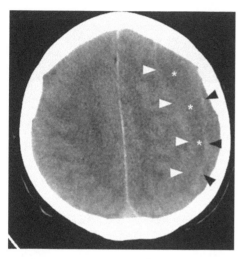

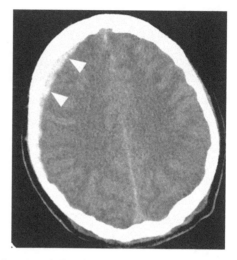

Case 1. A large collection is seen over the left cerebral convexity. This is slightly hypodense to grey matter (asterisk), suggesting that it is somewhat chronic, and exerts mass effect on the adjacent cerebral hemisphere (white arrowheads). Additionally, linear hyperdensity is also seen within the collection (black arrowheads), indicating more acute haemorrhage.
Diagnosis: Acute-on-chronic subdural haemorrhage.

Case 2. A shallow hyperdense collection is seen over the right frontal lobe (arrowheads).
Diagnosis: Acute subdural haemorrhage.

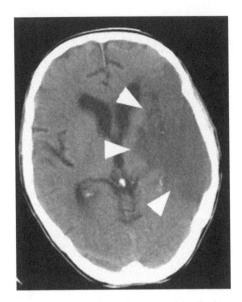

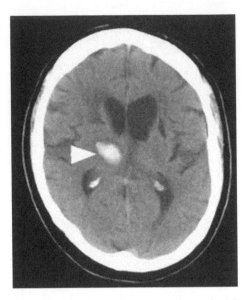

Case 3. Large area of low density, involving both grey and white matter, within the left middle cerebral artery territory (arrowheads). This does not demonstrate haemorrhagic transformation.
Diagnosis: Acute left middle cerebral artery territory infarct.

Case 4. Focal area of hyperdensity centred upon the right thalamus and lentiform nucleus (arrowhead).
Diagnosis: Acute parenchymal haemorrhage. This type of haemorrhage has a strong association with uncontrolled hypertension.

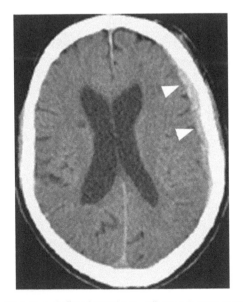

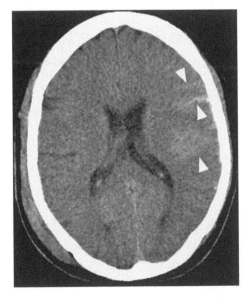

Case 5. A shallow hyperdense collection is seen over the left cerebral convexity (arrowheads).
Diagnosis: Acute subdural haemorrhage.

Case 6. Subtle linear hyperdensity is seen outlining several sulci within the left cerebral hemisphere (arrowheads).
Diagnosis: Acute subarachnoid haemorrhage.

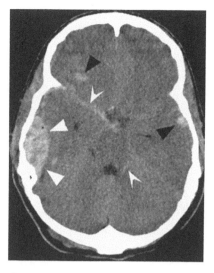

Case 7. Axial scan viewed on 'bone windows', demonstrating sharply marginated defects within the left occipital bone (arrowheads).
Diagnosis: Left occipital fracture.

Case 8.
  1. Hyperdense biconvex collection over the right temporal lobe (straight white arrowheads).
  2. Linear hyperdensity outlining the basal cisterns (curved arrowheads).
  3. Focal parenchymal hyperdensity (black arrowheads).
Diagnosis: Acute extradural haemorrhage with additional subarachnoid haemorrhage and parenchymal contusions.

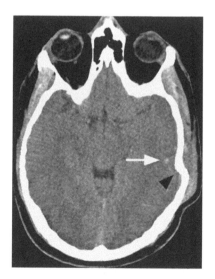

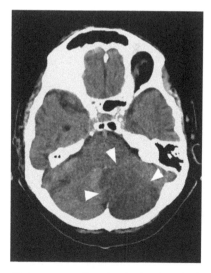

Case 9. Small focal area of hyperdensity seen within the left temporal lobe (arrow), with a small depression in the overlying left temporal bone (arrowhead). This should be assessed formally on bone windows.
Diagnosis: Depressed skull fracture with focal parenchymal contusion.

Case 10. Large area of low density, involving both grey and white matter, within the left cerebellar hemisphere (arrowheads). Associated compression of the fourth ventricle due to mass effect.
Diagnosis: Acute left cerebellar infarct.

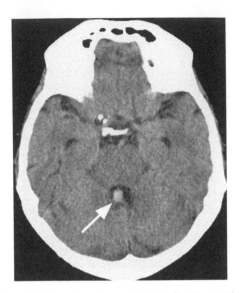

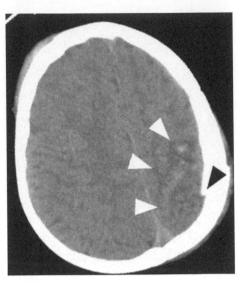

Case 11. Hyperdense focus within the fourth ventricle (arrow).
Diagnosis: Acute intraventricular haemorrhage.

Case 12. Small punctuate and linear areas of hyperdensity seen within the left superior parietal lobe, which is generally of reduced density (white arrowheads). In addition, there is a small 'step' in the inner table of the overlying parietal bone (black arrowhead). This should be formally assessed on bone windows.
Diagnosis: Left superior parietal contusions secondary to a depressed skull fracture.

Appendices

Appendix 1 ABCD^2 Scoring System

Table 7 ABCD^2 score for TIA risk assessment.

Criteria		Points
Age	Age $\geq$ 60	1
BP at assessment	Initial SBP $\geq$ 140 mmHg or DBP $\geq$ 90 mmHg	1
Clinical features	Unilateral weakness	2
	Speech disturbance	1
	Other symptoms	0
Duration	> 60 minutes	2
	10–59 minutes	1
	< 10 minutes	0
Diabetes		1

Total score is out of 7.

Those with a score of > 4 should be admitted to hospital for further assessment.

If score is < 4, outpatient referral to TIA clinic, or equivalent, could be considered based on clinical acumen.

Appendix 2 ROSIER Score

The aim of this assessment tool is to enable medical and nursing staff to differentiate patients with stroke and stroke mimics.

Assessment Date ☐☐☐☐☐☐ Time ☐☐☐☐

Symptom onset Date ☐☐☐☐☐☐ Time ☐☐☐☐

GGS E=☐ M=☐ V=☐ **BP** ☐☐ ***BM** ☐

* If BM < 3.5 mmol/l treat urgently and reassess once blood glucose normal

Has there been loss of consciousness or syncope?

Y (−1) ☐ N (0) ☐

Has there been seizure activity?

Y (−1) ☐ N (0) ☐

Is there a <u>NEW ACUTE</u> onset (or on awakening from sleep)?

I.	Asymmetric facial weakness	Y (+1) ☐	N (0) ☐
II.	Asymmetric arm weakness	Y (+1) ☐	N (0) ☐
III.	Asymmetric leg weakness	Y (+1) ☐	N (0) ☐
IV.	Speech disturbance	Y (+1) ☐	N (0) ☐
v.	Visual field defect	Y (+1) ☐	N (0) ☐

*Total Score _____ (−2 to +5)

Provisional diagnosis: ☐ Stroke ☐ Non-stroke (specify)_____

* Stroke is likely if total scores are > 0. Scores of </= 0 have a low possibility of stroke but not completely excluded.

Appendix 3 NICE Acute Stroke Flow Pathway

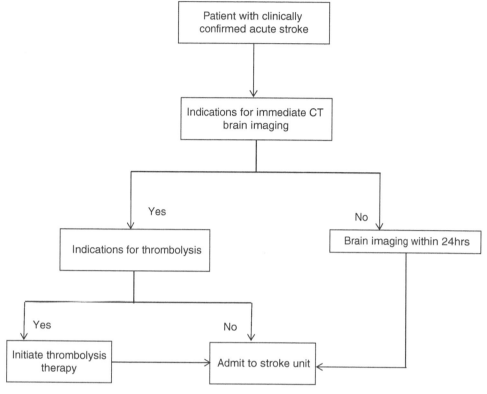

Figure 112 NICE Acute Stroke Flow Pathway.
http://pathways.nice.org.uk/pathways/stroke#path=view%3A/pathways/stroke/acute-stroke.xml&content=view-node%3Anodes-person-with-clinically-confirmed-acute-stroke

Appendix 4 Glasgow Coma Scale (GCS) Assessment

Eye response	Open spontaneously	4
	Open to verbal command	3
	Open to pain	2
	No response	1
Verbal response	Talking and orientated	5
	Confused/disorientated	4
	Inappropriate words	3
	Incomprehensible sounds	2
	No response	1
Motor response	Obeys commands	6
	Localises pain	5
	Flexion/withdrawal from pain	4
	Abnormal flexion	3
	Abnormal extension	2
	No response	1
TOTAL (GCS)		**Range 3–15**

Appendix 5 NICE Guideline for Adult CT Head

NICE National Institute for
Health and Care Excellence

Algorithm1:Selection of adults for CT head scan

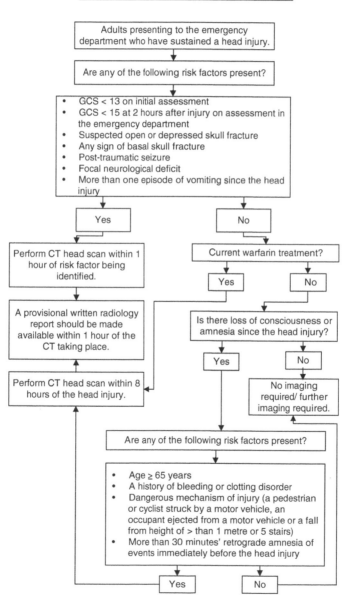

Appendix 6 NICE Guideline for Adult CT Neck

NICE National Institute for
Health and Care Excellence

Algorithm 3: Selection of adults for imaging of the cervical spine

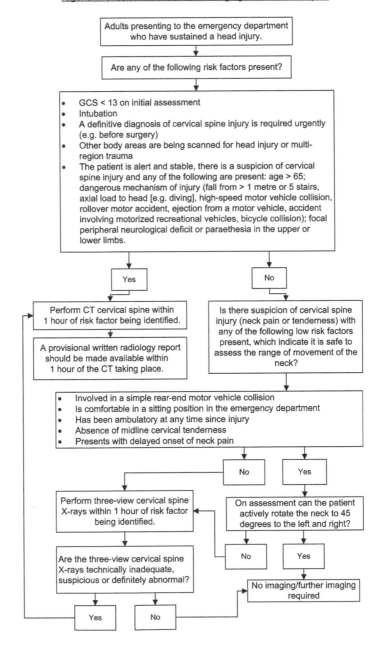

Appendix 7 NICE Guideline for Paediatric CT Head

NICE National Institute for
Health and Care Excellence

<u>**Algorithm 2: Selection of children for CT head scan**</u>

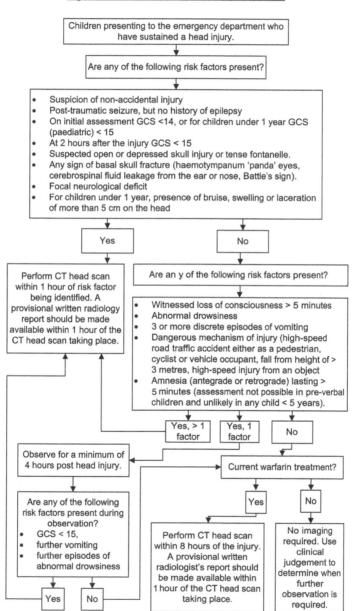

Children presenting to the emergency department who have sustained a head injury.

Are any of the following risk factors present?

- Suspicion of non-accidental injury
- Post-traumatic seizure, but no history of epilepsy
- On initial assessment GCS <14, or for children under 1 year GCS (paediatric) < 15
- At 2 hours after the injury GCS < 15
- Suspected open or depressed skull injury or tense fontanelle.
- Any sign of basal skull fracture (haemotympanum 'panda' eyes, cerebrospinal fluid leakage from the ear or nose, Battle's sign).
- Focal neurological deficit
- For children under 1 year, presence of bruise, swelling or laceration of more than 5 cm on the head

Yes

No

Perform CT head scan within 1 hour of risk factor being identified. A provisional written radiology report should be made available within 1 hour of the CT head scan taking place.

Are an y of the following risk factors present?

- Witnessed loss of consciousness > 5 minutes
- Abnormal drowsiness
- 3 or more discrete episodes of vomiting
- Dangerous mechanism of injury (high-speed road traffic accident either as a pedestrian, cyclist or vehicle occupant, fall from height of > 3 metres, high-speed injury from an object
- Amnesia (antegrade or retrograde) lasting > 5 minutes (assessment not possible in pre-verbal children and unlikely in any child < 5 years).

Yes, > 1 factor

Yes, 1 factor

No

Observe for a minimum of 4 hours post head injury.

Current warfarin treatment?

Are any of the following risk factors present during observation?
- GCS < 15,
- further vomiting
- further episodes of abnormal drowsiness

Yes

No

Yes

No

Perform CT head scan within 8 hours of the injury. A provisional written radiologist's report should be made available within 1 hour of the CT head scan taking place.

No imaging required. Use clinical judgement to determine when further observation is required.

Appendix 8 NICE Guideline for Paediatric CT Neck

NICE National Institute for Health and Care Excellence

Algorithm 4: Selection of children for imaging of the cervical spine

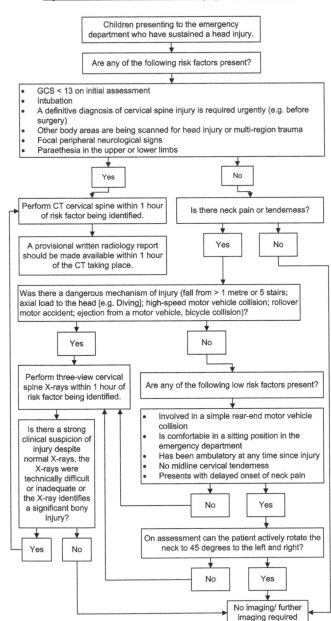

Appendix 9 Information Required Prior to Neurosurgical Transfer

- Before contacting the neurosurgeon, vital information and an updated clinical evaluation must be collated.
- The following list includes the minimum details that must be immediately available:
  - Referring hospital and named Consultant.
  - Patient demographics with hospital number.
  - Date and time of incident.
  - Time of admission.
  - History of event.
  - Physiological observations.

Table 9

Time	HR	BP	RR	O2 sat^n	GCS eye	GCS motor	GCS verbal	Right pupil reacts	Right pupil size	Left pupil reacts	Left pupil size
On arrival											
On transfer											

- CT scan/s at referring hospital   yes   No
- Result of CT scan of head:
- CT scan of neck/chest/abdomen/pelvis/face:
- Other injuries:
- Relevant past medical history:
- Allergies:
- Drug history:
- Last ingestion:
- Interventions: Airway: Guedel   ETT
  - Breathing: Spontaneous   IPPV
  - Circulation: Fluids   Urinary catheter
- Drugs given:
- Tetanus:
- Blood test results:
- X-match:
- Arterial blood gas:
- Urinalysis:
- Next of kin contact details: Notified: Yes   No
- Medical escort:
- Documentation for transfer: medical notes/Observation chart/Radiographs
- Receiving neurosurgeon:
- ETA:

Appendix 10 Differential Diagnosis for Intracerebral Lesions

Table 10 Calcified intracranial lesions.

Physiological	Choroid plexus, pineal
Neoplastic	Glioma: 5–10% (20% of astrocytomas) Meningioma: 15% calcify Metastases: occasionally calcify, particularly colon, breast and osteosarcoma Craniopharyngioma: 90% calcify in children, 40% in adults Chordoma: dense calcification in 50% adjacent to the clivus
Vascular	Aneurysm: 1% calcify AVMs: 15% calcify Chronic subdural haematoma: 1–5% calcify Chronic infarct
Infective	Abscess: calcification occurs late Tuberculoma: 1–5% calcify. Usually multiple Tuberculous meningitis Cysticercosis

Table 11 CT attenuation of cerebral masses (relative to normal brain).

Hyperdense	Isodense	Hypodense
Haematoma < 1 week	Haematoma 1–2 weeks	Haematoma > 2 weeks
Colloid cyst 50%	Colloid cyst 50%	Cysts: arachnoid, porencephalic, hydatid
Tuberculoma	Tuberculoma	Tuberculoma
Giant aneurysm	–	Pyogenic abscess
	Neoplasms	
Meningioma 95%	–	–
Primary lymphoma	–	–
Metastases 30%	Metastases 10%	Metastases 30%
Glioma 10%	Glioma 10%	Glioma
Ependymoma	–	–
Medulloblastoma 80%	–	–
Pituitary adenoma 25%	Pituitary adenoma 65%	–
Acoustic neuroma 5%	Acoustic neuroma 95%	
–	–	Prolactinoma
–	–	Haemangioblastoma
Papilloma	Chordoma	Lipoma
–	Pinealoma	Epidermoid
–	–	Dermoid
Craniopharyngioma (solid)	–	Craniopharyngioma